Cry but don't Panic

Janice Warner

DEDICATION

"Cry but don't Panic" is dedicated to brave-hearted people who battle cancer and other terminal illness. For many the 'C' word carries trauma as their lives will change. You may laugh today and cry tomorrow.

I have been there when my pastor-husband ministered at the bedside of a dying cancer patient. Through the years women in our congregations have come to me for encouragement when they first heard the 'C' word. They assumed their life was over. You may feel your future has been cancelled, but there is something called HOPE. Don't borrow fear from the unknown.

Cancer is a reality in my family. I have lost two siblings to cancer however my sister Ann has been a survivor of 4-stage breast cancer for 20+ years and to her I dedicate this book.

Only God knows why some survive and others do not. When it's your time to go you *will* go, whether by accident or disease. God offers you a generous portion of peace to carry you through this most traumatic ordeal– take it!

CONTENTS

Don't Panic

Occasionally into our lives
Adversity comes along.
We may ask ourselves,
"What have I done wrong?"

Why is it that frail humans
Are quick to take the blame?
Could it be natural causes
May have caused this pain?

Don't ever panic or give up
There's new hope just for you.
Jesus knows the pain you feel,
And He will see you through.

When you feel like crying
For a future unknown, go ahead.
Don't hold all the fear inside;
Talk it over with the Lord instead.

1

Why is this Happening to Me?

A chill shivered down my spine. Three life-threatening words pierced my consciousness with exquisite pain. I did not want to have this conversation with my doctor. The room suddenly felt cold and I pulled my cardigan tightly about me.

Dr. Nelson's deep-set brown eyes looked over his rimless glasses and into the depths of my being. He discerned I was unable to process the lab diagnosis and promised we would lick it together. I never dreamed I would one day hear the dreaded word CANCER.

He became silent for a few moments, measuring my reaction to the 'C' word. I was totally speechless. An alarm was going off inside me, hinting my time might soon be up. I stared straight ahead at the stark white walls of the doctor's office. Was this a bad dream?

Soon I was aware my doctor was still talking. However, his conversation had little chance of penetrating my brain. Instinctively I knew there was no degree of comfort in his words. Panic engulfed me.

Suddenly I felt very alone in a medical center humming with the activity of people walking about. My doctor was reassuring me that with the latest medical technology my chances for recovery were good. He repeated that he would be there for me and we would lick it together. His words fell on deaf ears. I knew deep in my heart life would never be the same again.

Nothing could have prepared me to receive this news. I had always believed if one takes care of his/her body chances of having cancer or any other serious disease were slim indeed. I had never entertained the thought there might be tumors growing on my ovaries. I thought the discomfort I had been experiencing was probably due to some minor thing that could be easily fixed. Cancer had never entered my thoughts.

There is no easy fix for ovarian cancer as symptoms lie silent while the disease grows. Researchers anticipate a breakthrough but when will it happen? When a cure finally breaks on the horizon, the discovery will bring much rejoicing to families worldwide.

It seemed like there was a two-ton elephant resting on my chest. My brain was paralyzed. I couldn't think. The walls of the medical office seemed to be squeezing in on me. I had to escape from this place that was causing me pain.

Dr. Nelson must have sensed my panic. He stood up, walked to my side and was about to place his hand on my shoulder, no doubt to reassure and comfort me. However, I rudely ignored him. In a flash, I jumped up and began to walk briskly out of his office. Outdoors, I breathed the fresh, sea air in gasps, wondering what I should do next.

Unlocking the car, I slumped down in the driver's seat mentally exhausted. My eyes were tightly closed so that

I couldn't see the movement of people coming and going to the medical facility. "Get ahold of yourself, girl," I was thinking. This was no time to fall apart. Surely there would be a way out of this maze.

My mind was trying to digest the thought of having cancer. How could I have cancer? Among my friends I was considered a "health nut" as I inspected and hand-picked all the food that came into our kitchen. I was conscious, not only of what I ate, but I felt responsible to serve nutritious, pesticide-free food to my family as well. Further, nearly every day I went jogging and spent time in exercise routines to keep fit. *Why is this happening to me?*

The lab report must certainly be mistaken! It couldn't be true! There's no way I could have cancer! Without a doubt my test results had been mixed up with someone else's in the lab. Perhaps more lab work would prove there had been an error. I wanted to cry, but tears were frozen deep inside me.

Slowly I began to drive in the direction of the beach, always a retreat from a hectic day. Powerful waves were coming ashore and washing up and over piles of tortured-looking driftwood strewn across the sandy beach. Glorious sunshine glistened on the crest of the busy waves. In and out, in and out, in exact rhythm, they soon coaxed me out of the car and onto the shoreline of the mighty Pacific Ocean.

Stepping out of my sandals I pressed my feet deep into the cool sand and stared hypnotically out across the water for a few moments. The power of the mighty sea was breathtaking! Aimlessly I walked along while the tide washed over my cool feet. Anyone looking on might think I was a carefree tourist strolling along a southern Oregon beach. There wasn't anything carefree about my attitude. If they could see inside me, they would discover a frenzy of churning like the undercurrent in the cold turquoise water stretched out before me.

As I meandered along the beach I finally came to a favorite place strewn with logs washed ashore in a storm. To the left was a cave. I knew it well for I had been there many times with my family. My husband Jeff and I enjoyed racing the children from the lifeguard station to the cave. The winner would be rewarded with a favorite treat at the ice cream shop overlooking the beach. If the lab report is accurate, it's possible I may have run my last race for ice cream.

I was fast slipping into despondency. I needed to get ahold of myself. Why was I so quick to assume a drastic conclusion regarding my life span when I had only surface information at this time?

There were a few smooth logs on the beach providing a place for me to sit down. This was a time for thinking things out. Gazing out upon the vast blue-green water, I watched the waves get higher and higher and then come crashing down in foamy patterns upon the sandy beach. The repetitive action held my attention. I could see forever and my thoughts suddenly turned to *time* and *eternity.*

At the age of 37, there was a lot of living yet to do. Sure, like most people I looked forward to Heaven someday, but not as a result of cancer – and not now! I wanted to grow old with wisdom, to make a meaningful contribution to my loved ones and friends. I hadn't yet done anything of particular note that might be mentioned at my memorial.

My children, Jeremy and Tina, were a big part of my life. I wanted to be there for them always. When they came in from school and called out, "Mom, I'm home," I wanted to be there to chat about their day and help with their homework. When they needed moral support and comfort, I wanted to be there to put my arms around them and shelter them from harm. I wanted to watch them grow up - go to college - and someday marry. I wanted the thrill of an exciting extended family, holding precious grandchildren in my arms. Was I being selfish?

If Jeff came home discouraged because a special project at work wasn't going smoothly, I wanted to be there to listen and encourage him. When he laid work out on the dining room table that kept him up until midnight or later, I wanted to be there to distract him: to sneak up and put my arms around him or offer him a glass of sparkling iced lemonade to refresh him. Was I being selfish?

Jeff was the ideal husband. He was handsome. He had winsome ways. He was caring and thoughtful and just plain fun to be with. His beautiful smiling eyes captivated my attention the first time we met - and they hadn't changed. Jeff and I had enjoyed 14 wonderful years together, but that's not nearly enough to fulfill all our plans and dreams.

Feeling I had been handed a death sentence, my mind was racing with crazy, disconnected thoughts. How would Jeff get along without me if cancer should take my life? Would he marry again and bring a stranger into our home to raise our children? How would Jeremy and Tina react to a new mom? Would she love them as if they were her own? Is it possible there really could be a good substitute for a birth mother? A senseless twinge of jealousy was creeping into my thoughts. I needed to be more positive and not be worrying about things un-known over which I certainly had no control.

The children and I had been great pals, with fun shop-ping trips for athletic shoes or hair ribbons or a new dress. Jeremy's ballgames and Tina's weekly piano lessons were important to both Jeff and me. We were a close-knit family that made room for recreation that could be enjoyed by all four of us. Our family theme had always been 'togetherness.'

Jeff had recently become executive vice president in the company. We enjoyed a good lifestyle. He provided an excellent income so that I had never worked outside the home since the children were born. It had been a delight to be a stay-at-home mom.

I was the exception among my friends as I loved being a housewife and homemaker, creating a peaceful retreat for my family after a busy day at school or work. When I held our first child in my arms, I was smitten with motherly love. It would be impossible for me to go back to my chosen career as a fashion designer. I wanted to experience the joy of being a full-time mother to these precious gifts from God.

How could I have cancer and maybe die and leave them? I couldn't! I wouldn't! My emotions took over and I jumped to my feet, threw up my hands in frustration and shouted to the heavens, *"Why is this happening to me?"* I don't know what I expected, but I didn't hear the voice of the Lord thunder forth. There was only a deafening silence as I stood on a lonely southern Oregon beach.

The powerful ocean was spread out before me. The only evidence of life was that of busy seagulls that never seemed to spend more than a second in any one place.

To be alone on the beach was quite unusual. Normally beachcombers and mommies with little toddlers would be scooping up shells and playing in the sand. At this time there was nobody in sight who might disturb my train of thought. I wished there might be someone I could talk to, share my inner pain and perhaps get some encouragement. This was by far the most traumatic and frightening time I had ever known and I needed a comforting shoulder to cry on.

There were serious things I needed to think about in order to make decisions. I'm not sure, but I think my doctor mentioned chemotherapy when I shut him out and left his office. It's difficult to decide today if I would choose to undergo chemo. I had known people who opted NOT to undergo chemo treatment in order to have a somewhat better quality of life for the days or months they may have. Some of my friends had chemo which was successful in putting them into remission. Others had chemo and suffered from almost constant nausea and vomiting and were reduced to a skeleton frame.

How could I decide what to do? If one could know at the outset chemo would be effective, the obvious choice would be to submit to the treatment. However, if one could know chemo would fail while cancer continued invading the body, the obvious decision might be to reject the treatment along with side-effects it often causes. I would have to make the decision regarding chemo later. Am I going to die?

- How much time do I have?

- How will cancer affect my family?

- Will my friends be supportive?

- Can cancer be reversed?

- What should I do now?

The weight of the 'C' word was crushing the breath out of me. I felt I was being pulled deep into the ocean by tormenting waves washing ashore and taking anything in its path out to sea.

I began walking in quick strides along the damp sand. *"How do I break this awful news to my family, when it's crushing me"* I wondered. Handling bad news gracefully had never been one of my talents.

The initial shock of being told you have cancer is impossible to describe. It is unbelievable. You deny it, refuse it and are positive there must be a mistake! It cannot be true. In my heart I knew I needed to have a positive attitude toward an aggressive attack on the disease, however I wasn't sure I could be strong enough for the entire ordeal. Perhaps if I could talk with someone else who may be in the same situation as I, it would be a little easier to understand what may lie ahead.

Reader, hearing the 'C' word is traumatic to say the least, but it certainly does not signify you must begin to plan your memorial. Continue in your current day-to-day routine as long as you can. If you walk several times a week, keep it up. If you are a teacher, a secretary, or work in a factory, continue in your vocation as long as you can. At some point, you will need to advise your supervisor of the situation as there will be appointments to keep with your physician, etc.

You don't need to advertise to other employees that you are undergoing cancer treatment. They will discover this in time anyway. Go pleasantly about your work. Work is good, too, as it will take your mind off the thought of cancer. This is no time to 'shut down.'

You have much to live for. Many good books and magazines deal with cancer. Read them to become more knowledgeable on how others cope with the disease. Survivors are all around us and you may soon be added to that number.

Panicking will cripple you from the normal day-to-day experience you want. If you panic, there may be many anxious and restless days and nights. Happiness is contagious. When you are happy it spills over onto those around you.

Gazing up at the sky, seagulls soared above the water, graceful and carefree in flight. Oh that I might be so carefree. Watching the mighty waves as they crashed onto the rocky shoreline before me, I felt a new sense of the impending storm that would soon envelope me. I also knew I wasn't alone as every day thousands just like me will hear the 'C' word.

For some, the life-threatening words YOU HAVE CANCER may terrorize their spirits. Others receive the news in a matter-of-fact fashion and go about their daily routine as usual. Still others will hold this news inside, refusing to discuss it. I was only one among many brave men and women afflicted with terminal illness. How do they cope with devastating news when their lives take an undesirable direction? Do they look up to the Lord, our maker, and trust Him for healing?

It had been over an hour since I had escaped from the doctor's office. Perhaps I had gained enough composure to go home and face my family. However I knew deep in my heart I wasn't yet able to talk about the 'C' word. I must wait for the very best time. In fact, it might be a good idea to wait for additional lab work to be processed to be sure Dr. Nelson's diagnosis is correct before I share the idea of my having cancer with my family. Perhaps it would be best to keep Dr. Nelson's diagnosis between him and me for awhile.

Inspiration

"Turn yourself to me and have mercy upon me
for I am desolate and afflicted. The troubles of my heart
have enlarged; oh, bring me out of my distresses."
Psalm 25:16

Application

Suddenly I don't know if there will be another tomorrow. My future is looking bleak; my sight has no clarity after hearing the 'C' word from the doctor.

How can this be happening to me? I am angry for I have taken good care of my body. I am frustrated because I am in the prime of life with a wonderful family. This is a burden too heavy to carry.

My orderly life has taken an unexpected bend in the road. What should I do now? Will our annual family vacation be cancelled because I am ill?

"Please God, talk to me. I need your guidance as I begin to walk through this maze. Please send rays of sunlight to break through the fog of anxiety and self-pity I'm stuck in. I need a measure of peace to carry me through this totally unexpected and difficult time."

✢✢✢

For dinner I made a meatloaf, baked potatoes, and created a green salad which was thoroughly enjoyed by my
family. As usual, we sat at the table chatting about the
day's activities. Later as I was loading the dishwasher
Jeff sneaked up and put his arms around me. "What did
you do today?" he whispered in my ear. "Oh, not
much," was my faint reply. He turned me around to face
him. "As I recall you had an appointment with the doctor. How did it go?" This caught me totally off-guard. I
tried to turn my face from Jeff, but he could see the
moisture glistening in my eyes. Then he drew me close
and I could feel his face against my wet cheeks.

In a flash, Jeff picked me up and carried me from the
kitchen to the family room. "The dishes can wait. Let's
have a little talk." (Jeff already knew about my visit with
Dr. Nelson as the doctor contacted him when I abruptly
walked out of his office earlier in the day.) Suddenly it
seemed all the calm I had gained walking along the
beach was vanishing and I had a deep, deep longing for
sympathy from my husband. Frozen tears from deep
within me began to melt just a little.

With much tenderness Jeff began, "Hon, I know you don't want to talk about your visit to the doctor but we need to face the reality of the lab report. Being told you have cancer is terribly frightening. I'm frightened too. Dr. Nelson had a long talk with me today and he assured me you will have the best treatment there is." I spoke up quickly, "What do you mean I will have the best of treatment? Do you remember the agony Jackie endured when struggling to overcome ovarian cancer? Now I have the same cancer!"

"Yes, I remember Jackie's difficult battle, but this is now several years down the road and research has made better treatments available for patients," Jeff responded hopefully as he stroked my hair. "You may breeze right through therapy to remission in a short time."

"I'll be by your side all the way," Jeff continued. "If you agree, Dr. Nelson wants to refer you to Dr. Unruh, a skilled oncologist at the Cancer Center in the city. He feels Dr. Unruh, will provide the care you need to come through this ordeal. How do you feel about it?" At that moment in time there was no way I could give an opinion to Jeff as it was too personal for me. He continued,

"We will not give up and, most of all, we aren't going to panic. We trust in God." I could agree with Jeff on this point: I would keep a positive thought. At least for a few moments, my faith in God was set in concrete.

Out of curiosity, Jeremy and Tina would occasionally walk by and peek into the room. Sensing something was wrong they finally decided to join us. Jeff was great. He explained to them that "Mom needs our help right now. She has just learned she is very ill." Jeremy was quick to blurt out, "What's wrong Mom? Is it serious?" "Yes son," Jeff cut in, "Mom saw the doctor today and learned she has cancer." Almost in unison the children murmured, "Cancer?" They also panicked at hearing the 'C' word.

Jeremy and Tina came quickly to my side. Tina wrapped her little arms around my neck and began sobbing quietly. She was afraid, as I had been at the moment Dr. Nelson said the 'C' word to me. Jeff encircled Tina and Jeremy in his long strong arms to comfort them. He explained I would be under the care of a skilled oncologist in the city who would give me the best of care. Then he reminded us of Mrs. Savage, a neighbor who had been diagnosed with cancer several years earlier. After a year or more of treatments, her cancer was in remission and she was still a healthy survivor.

It was evident our children had a lot of unspoken questions. The mere thought of cancer often sends panic into one's consciousness and my children were no exception. Jeff mentioned we would stick together to get me through this ordeal. We must depend upon the Lord for new strength every day. Clearing his throat, he continued, "I know how hard this may be, but we have always trusted God and this is no different from any other situation." Jeff read the 23rd Psalm from the Bible.

Psalm 23

The Lord is my shepherd. I shall not want. He maketh me lie down in green pastures. He leadeth me beside the still waters. He restoreth my soul. He leadeth me in the paths of righteousness for His name's sake.

Yea though I walk through the valley of the shadow of death I will fear no evil for thou art with me. Thy rod and Thy staff, they comfort me.

Thou preparest a table before me in the presence of mine enemies; Thou anointest my head with oil; my cup runneth over.

Surely goodness and mercy shall follow me all the days of my life and I will dwell in the house of the Lord forever.

It was necessary to get away where I could vent my emotions without making a fool of myself.

Alone in the bathroom the chilly ice that had formed around my emotions melted like butter on a hot stove. I was crying for myself. I was crying for Jeff. I was crying for the children. Their prayers had touched me. I could not control feeling drowned in the overall implications of the day.

Soon Jeff was rapping on the bathroom door. "Honey, are you alright," he wanted to know. Somehow I managed to blubber some response and he sensed my need for privacy and slipped away. I was thankful the Lord had given me such a thoughtful and caring husband. I was blessed.

While I have stood beside the bed of friends who fought cancer, the thought of the disease touching me had always seemed remote. Now Cancer had become very personal. I would engage in battle against the disease but I knew I would *not* have to fight alone for the Lord would surely take care of me. I thanked the Lord for the boundless love and compassion He shows toward those who put their trust in Him.

Though I did not know what God's plan for my life might be, I knew His love and care would sustain me. With my faith in God and my adoring husband by my side, I could get through this ordeal. Also I felt certain my close friends would surround me with much-needed support. What are friends for anyway?

Little did I know then there would be many ups and downs in my emotional makeup during the next twelve or eighteen months. Just when I thought I had control of the situation, everything would fall apart. I vacillated between faith and anxiety constantly. It was like being on an old fashioned teeter-totter, only I wasn't having any fun!

> Reader, remember, Jesus knows how you feel. He sees every teardrop that moistens your eyes. He knows when you are afraid and anxious regarding your future. He wants to take the anxiety and fear from you and give you peace. He wants you to be free from any tormenting thoughts that may come against you as you lie upon your bed, sleepless, worrying about tomorrow. Ask Him for peace and trust in Him.

Do you know the Lord so that you may rely upon His promises? Do you believe Jesus will give you peace in the midst of the storm if you trust in Him? From personal experience, I know how difficult it is to abandon one's future to the Lord and leave it there. There are times we seem to need to dwell on negatives that happen in our lives, whatever they may be.

Rather than leave our burdens at the foot of the cross, we sometimes take them back and carry them. The wondrous truth is Jesus took our burdens at Calvary when He became the ultimate sacrifice for our sins!

The next morning I made breakfast for Jeremy and Tina and sat chatting with them before they left for school. There was no mention of cancer as we talked excitedly about their anticipated activities of the day. I didn't want them to be burdened with the thought that mom was diagnosed with cancer. They needed to study and interact with classmates as usual, without distractions.

Soon the children were on the bus and I poured a cup of my favorite breakfast tea and made myself comfortable on the patio. The warm morning sun was welcome on my back. Gazing out upon the lake, and listening to the gentle ebb and flow of the water at the shoreline I felt peace on this most perfect day.

I loved our location, somewhat secluded from the main street of our little town. There was no traffic here and our closest neighbor was an acre away. It was quite a change from busy city life. Five years ago when we bought our home, Jeff had purchased ten acres of prime land bordering the lake and our property in this sleepy little mill town. Cedar, pine and fir trees flourished in abundance. Colorful rhododendrons and azaleas dotted the landscape among the lush, green forest. What a beautiful place to live!

Our property was at the edge of Garrison Lake and per-haps half a mile from the Pacific Ocean. This sleepy little town had a number of beaches where one could walk along the sand and surf, hunting agates, drift-wood and other treasures from the sea. When we dis-covered this property, we felt especially blessed to be so near the ocean and at the edge of a lake with our own boat dock.

A strip of lawn not more than 20 feet wide separated our house from the bank. Ducks nested there, leaving tracks all along the grassy strip. They were a messy crew, but the privilege of living on the lake made up for the effort of cleaning up after these interesting creatures that never tired of waddling along the lake shore quacking noisily.

My flower beds provided special color and the fragrance of cut flowers was common in our house during the spring and summer months. I heaved a deep sigh, at peace with the tranquil scene laid out before me.

Events of yesterday seemed somewhat unreal. Had I really been in Dr. Nelson's office? Had he really told me I have cancer? Had he really discussed the urgency for surgery and follow-up chemo?

Things were moving too fast! It wasn't difficult to acknowledge the need for surgery, because the tumors must be removed before the cancer spreads. However I was having a mental battle with the thought of undergoing chemotherapy. Couldn't people see this was a decision I wasn't ready to make at the time? Why was the doctor asking me to make a decision so soon? I needed time to think things out more clearly.

Mere words cannot describe the helplessness of the situation. It was as if I was on a runaway train, picking up speed on the downgrade. I felt only a tiny bit of confidence that I would return to health, knowing there had been little research on ovarian cancer and remembering my dear friend, Jackie.

The small measure of calm assurance gathered last evening was fading. My eyes were misting and I choked to keep from crying. Cat nuzzled close to me, trying in her own way to comfort me. However, this seemed to be a time when there couldn't be any lasting comfort. I had to vent my anxiety and fear through my tears. How would I ever reclaim the measure of joy I had known?

Sipping the delicious tea I was wondering how one day I could be enjoying a carefree lifestyle and the next be stopped by flashing lights and danger signs indicating the bridge was washed out on *my* road of life. Surrounded by high water, there seemed no place to go. I was drowning in my sorrow.

As a Christian, I knew I should turn my seemingly help-less situation over to the Lord. He had never failed me. He had always been faithful. Why was it so difficult for me to trust Him to bring this excruciating personal trial to a good conclusion? It was important that I try to control my emotions or I would not be any good to myself or my family as we entered this new saga together.

I knew Jesus could do the impossible. I knew He could speak two little words, "Be healed" and cancer would leave my body. I tried to trust Him and be at peace. Every morning of my adult life I had asked the Lord to lead me and have His way in my life. I knew He would take care of me as I walked down this new path.

Never before had I faced an uncertain future. Though surrounded by the enduring love of my husband and children, I felt somewhat alone. I was beginning to feel the pressure of the two-ton elephant again.

I went into the house to retrieve my Bible, always a source of inspiration and faith. Returning to the patio, I discovered Cat had curled up in my patio chair. I lifted her and let her curl up in my lap again as I resumed my place in the warming sun.

Turning the pages of the Bible, a particular verse caught my eye. In Matthew 28:18 these words were spoken by Jesus after his resurrection: *"All power is given unto me, both in heaven and in earth."* What powerful words! I read this verse over and over again in order to absorb the full meaning. Finally I began to realize that Jesus IS in control of every situation, whether in heaven or in earth. And *He has the power to change any and all circumstances.* I felt reassured that Jesus did have full control in my life. I knew He had not put cancer upon me. <u>Sickness and disease are a result of the original sin in the garden of Eden.</u>

"In thee, O Lord, do I put my trust: let me never be put to confusion. Deliver me in thy righteousness and cause me to escape: incline thine ear unto me and save me."
Psalm 71:1

While I did not know what the future would hold for me or how many days or months or even years I may have I decided to trust the Lord for all my needs. I was hoping

I could hold onto this trust and not start doubting again in a few hours or tomorrow.

I needed balance in my life both today and every day into the future.

> I know Jesus has a master plan for my life. I must trust in Him and not waver.

Actually I had been asking the Lord to mold me into a vessel He could use. Is it possible this trial may be part of His master plan? I was feeling somewhat encouraged and began to thank the Lord for helping me see a little more clearly through the fog of discouragement.

The telephone rang and I quickly ran into the house to answer it. Pastor Murphy was calling to let me know he would like to meet with us in our home tonight. It seemed apparent Jeff had talked with our pastor about my diagnosis and he was coming over to encourage me and pray with me for healing.

It was like Jeff to do that. Jeff is a member of the Church board and close to Pastor Murphy. He and I were always involved in some church activity. I promised to make Pastor's favorite dessert for the occasion.

I tidied up a bit before baking the Mile-High Orange Cake pastor loves so much. This activity took my mind off myself, a good thing. Soon I was humming a little chorus of by-gone days, *"He careth for you; He careth for you. In sunshine or shadow, He careth for you."* (author unknown). Over and over I hummed this little chorus while recalling a verse from 1 Peter 5:7: *"Casting all your care upon Him for He careth for you."* Wonderful peace began to flood my soul. I made a commitment to stop fretting and cast my care on Jesus.

> *Reader, Jesus knows the pain you feel. He sees you on the mountain top and He knows when you're in the valley. Because He cares for you, you may put your trust in Him without doubting. Jesus suffered both mental and physical anguish as He hung upon Calvary's cross. He suffered for you and for me so our sins may be forgiven when we come to Him in repentance. That's how much He cares for YOU!*

I was feeling thankful for God's care and His wonderful goodness. I was thankful the Lord had made the ultimate sacrifice for my sins so that I might have eternal life if I confessed my sins (and I have done that). My heart was filled with thanks for God's everlasting love and His unfailing faithfulness. I was feeling joyous, full of hope and trust. It was wonderful to be free of anxiety.

The pastor arrived, his cheery self. He was well loved by the people of his parish, partly because of his upbeat personality. There was never anything in his way. With faith in Jesus every mountain could be climbed, every river could be crossed. God would make a way where there was no way. As I sat across the room from him, I realized how much I needed to hear encouraging words at this difficult time.

After a brief chitchat, pastor began to talk directly to me. He said, "I know how difficult it is to cope with the reality that you have cancer. It's not as easy to deal with as a broken bone that can be set and healed. However, there's no reason to panic as medical research continues to develop new and better treatment.

Further, you can have the peace of God in your soul as you fight this bitter disease. Rely on the Word to give you strength. Don't hesitate to talk to God about your feelings. He knows the pain you feel about an unknown future. No one understands like Jesus. Through this fiery trial you will learn to trust Him completely."

Pastor read some comforting scripture. One verse from Psalm 34:15 reads: *"The eyes of the Lord are on the righteous and his ears are open to their cry."* This was a positive and encouraging scripture which gave me hope. He told me the Lord would give me strength to endure this new venture down an unknown path. Further, he said pastor's door is always open whenever I may feel the need for encouragement and strength to go another mile. If I'm not feeling like getting out of the house, all I need do is call his office and he will come for a ministerial visit. It was good to know he would be available to lift me up when I might be down. Pastor led in prayer, asking the Lord to touch me with healing power.

Jeff's cousin, Eddie arrived the next day from Baltimore where he is employed by the U.S. Postal Service. The trauma of current events had caused me to forget his visit until he was standing at the door. It was always a treat to have Eddie in our home. He was a cut-up, able to keep the children laughing.

Jeremy and Tina weren't home from school when Eddie arrived. I invited him in and we sipped iced tea and chatted about family happenings since we had last seen each other.

Jeff and Eddie seemed to be total opposites. Jeff was 6' 3" tall with broad shoulders and a slim build; Eddie was not over 5' 7" and somewhat 'rounded out.' The little hair he had was dark. Eddie was a sweet, generous person, a delight to have around.

Four years ago Eddie's wife lost her battle with leukemia. Since then, he had buried himself in his work. Eddie and his wife had not been blessed with children and there weren't any other children in the family as young as our two, so Eddie doted on them.

When he heard the school bus coming down the street, Eddie stepped out to the front steps to greet them with thoughtfully chosen gifts. He gave Jeremy a Civil War game he could play with a friend across the street. Tina received an adorable 18-inch Japanese doll complete with a silk wardrobe. Eddie remembered her interest in collecting dolls of various cultures. These treasured gifts took precedence over homework that evening.

We enjoyed dessert on the patio where we could look out across the lake. There was interesting conversation as we tried to catch up on family news. It was a sunset to remember. The rays of the sun stretched across the horizon, painting clouds in pink and peach hues. Colorful reflections lay upon the surface of the placid lake.

Eddie and Jeff remained by the lake enjoying the cool gentle breeze while I went into the house to tuck the children into bed. I rejoined them to hear Eddie telling Jeff he had recently been diagnosed with colon cancer. His treatment was scheduled to begin in a few days. It was good to know Eddie's doctor felt he had an excellent chance of full recovery. Jeff had two persons close to him fighting cancer. Though he always seemed to be a tower of strength, I couldn't help but wonder what his private thoughts might have been during this test of his faith.

Partners in marriage support each other through thick or thin, through adversity or good times, through sickness or health. One's love doesn't diminish when life's high-way takes a sudden bend.

Friend, the love of family should grow stronger when one party is hurting. A spouse should do all he/she can to make the afflicted comfortable. The patient needs to draw encouragement and a sense all will soon return to normal from a spouse.

Some families grow apart when one spouse has a life-threatening illness. This is a mystery to me. How can a husband or wife abandon a spouse in the most difficult crisis of their life? Pity the man or woman who is unfaithful to their marriage vows when their partner is desperately fighting for life.

Others, too, should run to the side of their friends when they receive traumatic news of a serious disease from which they may not recover. How can you distance yourself from one you've cherished as a friend for many years? They are waiting for a phone call or knock on the door. As a special gesture, you might pick a few blooms from your garden for your ill friend. Could you find time to shop for groceries, or mail letters, and do other errands for your friend? This is what friends are for.

Inspiration

"I will lift up my eyes to the hills from whence cometh my help. My help cometh from the Lord who made heaven and earth."

Psalm 121:1

Application

God is mighty. God is powerful. He flung the worlds into space and holds them there with His hand. Realizing the tremendous power of my maker, I was aware of how very small my present need was. And I also knew God cared about me. He would carry me through this agonizing trial.

I was waging a battle for my life and there was comfort in knowing my help comes from the Lord. All good things come from Him. He will be my source of strength as I struggle to overcome cancer.

God who plotted the course of the stars in the heavens is looking after me with tender care. My trust is in Him.

2

An Important Decision

Dr. Unruh, a noted oncologist at the Cancer Center in the city was delightful. I had expected him to be quiet and reserved – all business. He instantly put me at ease. After introductions he suggested we walk to the Poetic Garden where we could discuss my treatment.

The garden evidenced great care in landscaping design. It was divided into a rock garden, dahlia garden, rose garden, etc. White wrought iron tables and chairs were scattered about. Short poems of hope etched on banners by recovering patients were hung where they could easily be read by others to lift their spirits.

We sat down and Dr. Unruh asked how I was feeling. He seemed to be analyzing my anxiety level. He acknowledged the trauma a patient must feel at the onset of discovery. He did not minimize the pain of hearing the 'C' word. His theme seemed to be 'attitude.' Dr. Unruh said 95 percent of recovery is based on good positive expectancy for healing.

He had reviewed my medical records forwarded by Dr. Nelson and felt because I was in excellent health my chance for recovery was excellent. My spirits immediately lifted. There was hope!

Soon we were discussing treatment, setting appointments and then it was time to return home. Walking back to his office, the doctor stressed the Cancer Center would provide for my medical, nutritional, physical, psychological and spiritual needs.

Dr. Unruh promised me the very best of care. What was he talking about, I wondered? Best of care? If chemo was the best he could offer, then perhaps there was little hope for my recovery. I had read about the results of chemo. And I remembered my best friend, Jackie, who suffered many months and in the end we lost her in spite of treatment.

After a few months of chemotherapy Jackie's strength began to diminish. She would sleep all night and lay on the couch most of the day. Soon she began to have bouts of vomiting, unable to keep food on her stomach. Family and friends were faithful to bring nourishing dishes to her but as the cancer progressed she made little effort to taste them. In the final stages she was too weak to feed herself if she wanted to eat. Wretched vomiting continued and once she was confined to bed, it was an ordeal to get to the bathroom.

For obvious reasons, Jackie chose not to wear her wig while lying in bed. Or, as mentioned earlier, her bed-clothes may have needed changed. When family or friends would rap on the door of her room she would call out in a weak voice, "Just a minute" until she could get her wig on. As the disease progressed she didn't have the strength to reach the hairpiece and would simply call out, "Don't come in. You can't come in." Because of her personal pride she was depriving herself of much-needed friendship and care.

Jackie was dedicated to her grandchildren. She wanted to be sure they lacked for nothing. She had a mind-set to 'gift' them even when there was no occasion for it. Jackie never tired of taking her grandchildren to fun places. Surely these perceptive children knew something was wrong with their grandmother they loved dearly. They must have wondered why she came to visit less often and why they were no longer invited for weekend visits.

They pestered their parents with questions such as, "Why are Grandma's hands stiff and crippled? Why is Grandma using a cane? Grandma said she doesn't have any feeling left in her feet and legs. Why is Grandma getting so skinny and wrinkled? What has happened to her? Isn't there anything the doctors can do for Grandma so she can get well?"

I shall never forget sitting in the passenger seat one afternoon while Jackie drove to the store. It was almost impossible for her to negotiate the curves on the country road. Fortunately there wasn't any traffic at that time. Jackie explained there was little feeling in her hands and she was also losing feeling in her feet and legs.

When I inquired about it, she replied the doctor said it was a side-effect of chemo.

Once when Jackie felt too weak to drive to the doctor's office, I offered to drive her downtown. It had been several weeks since I had seen her and I was shocked to discover how thin she had become. Always a proud woman, she tried to resist assistance getting into the car, but I too am a strong-willed person and she needed help, so I got her settled in the passenger seat. Glancing at her from the corner of my eye, I detected a little smile and knew she had appreciated the help after all.

The doctor gave Jackie a supply of nutritionally balanced liquid food, but my friend had always been a picky eater with very definite dislikes and she told me she "wasn't going to change her eating habits now." Family and friends failed in their efforts to encourage Jackie to maintain a good diet, including Vitamin C. It hurt to watch this beautiful, active person I had known and loved for so many years drop from 138 pounds to a skeleton.

Looking into the mirror each day, Jackie, who had always been proud of her beauty, would stare at a face that was no more than a mass of deep wrinkles. Her eyes had become dark, deep holes in her face. Though she joked and called herself "Packy" (for a baby elephant born at the Portland zoo many years prior), we all knew she hurt deeply at the physical changes taking place. This was an event my take-charge friend could not change – it was out of her control.

I kept in touch with Jackie. Prior to her passing, I spent many hours with her family as they stood at her bedside. Their care for her was evident as they gently stroked their mother's arm and whispered "I love you mom." It was heartbreaking to watch them grieve. It seemed so hopeless and senseless too, losing a vibrant, energetic woman to cancer. All of us knew she was holding onto life with a vengeance because she couldn't bear to part from her lovely children and grandchildren. I, too, couldn't bear the thought of losing my wonderful friend.

Jackie was a Christian. Once I picked up her worn Bible from the hospital nightstand and a scrap of paper dropped onto the floor. She had written, "For me to live is Christ, and to die is gain." Jackie knew if she should not recover she would be in the presence of the Lord.

I hadn't meant to go on and on about my friend, Jackie, so much but this was my first time to witness the death of anyone with cancer. The things I saw were not pretty and they were etched on my mind. Having seen the result of chemo I determined that if I should ever be faced with a decision regarding chemotherapy, I would elect *not* to undergo treatment and perhaps have a better quality of life.

Once when visiting Jackie at the hospital I followed her doctor into the hall and asked him why he had prescribed chemo since its side-effects had crippled her. His stoic reply was "We have to give cancer patients some hope and chemotherapy seems to do that."

Now with Jackie in mind, I may repeat myself over and over again and choose to reject chemotherapy. However Dr. Unruh prevailed, making me believe I must take the treatments for my family's sake if for no other reason. He told me chemo had improved in the past few years since Jackie underwent therapy and he felt I should at least give it a try.

Chemotherapy began. It treated me better than I had thought it might. True, after each treatment, I was weak for several days. I would sleep all night and get up in the morning and make breakfast as usual for the children. I did need to lie down during the day, but I was able to continue my household chores, go to the grocery store, keep the budget and pay bills for quite some time. As chemo treatments continued month after month and my energy diminished, Jeff took over these basic duties.

I put a great deal of effort into spending time with my two children before they boarded the bus for school each day. It was interesting to listen to them talk about their teachers.

Weeks became months and chemo continued. After five or six months my strength became weakness. I wasn't getting better. Family and friends could see that my health was failing. I told my doctor the chemo wasn't helping and I'd like to discontinue it in order to have a better quality of life. Jeff and Dr. Unruh had a conference and the consensus was that the therapy should not be discontinued.

A Secret Place

There is a secret place where one may hide
      from life's storms.
There is a secret place where one may trust
      and not be afraid.
In this secret place the Lord awaits,
      our deliverer.
Under His mighty arms we may rest secure,
      free from all harm.
Oh, come aside and rest in the secret place
      our Lord has made.
Though pressed with care you will find Him there
      in the secret place.
There is a secret place where there's not a trace
      of fear or harm.
Under His mighty wings your heart can sing:
      You know no care.
Oh, come aside and rest; do not be distressed
      and hopeless.
The Lord will dry your tears, take away your fear
      and meet you in the secret place.

Though Jeff had now assumed responsibility for grocery shopping and paying monthly bills, there really wasn't anyone to assume the job of cooking and keeping our house clean and tidy. When I thought about the neglect in keeping our place up I became depressed. Ours had always been a home with a place for everything and everything in its place.

Due to my limitations, our family managed the best we could without complaining. There was nothing we could do about it and we all seemed to accept it.

Jeff stocked the freezer with microwave dinners and instructed Jeremy and Tina in their preparation for eve-nings he had to work late or would be out of town. He also tried to keep some kind of dessert in the kitchen for a little taste of sweetness while there was nobody to do baking.

At first the children considered microwave food a treat, but before long they were wishing for salads, fried chicken, spaghetti, warm biscuits and muffins from the oven - and all the good meals they had been used to when I had kept the kitchen humming.

Pastor Murphy and his wife Allison came to the rescue. They had dropped by at suppertime one evening and discovered Tina trying to make a vegetable salad. Our pastor's wife organized a group of women from our large church who would prepare a complete evening meal on a rotating basis for us. It was a generous gesture and much appreciated.

Cancer continued to advance and I continued to get weaker. The house continued to show signs of definite neglect. It became more and more apparent that we needed a housekeeper. Again the pastor's wife recruited a couple of ladies from the women's group at church who came once a week to vacuum, change bedding, do laundry, and clean the kitchen and bathrooms. They were absolutely wonderful! Jeremy and Tina were especially excited about help with housework. I can never thank my family and friends enough for the support they gave me at that difficult time.

As time went on, a side-effect of chemo developed: stiffness in my arms, making it difficult to slip a knit top or sweater over my head. I hadn't said anything about it, but Jeff, being the observant man he was, bought me several loose fitting shifts. I could just slip them on and zip them up. With a pair of terry scuffs on my feet and my cane in hand, I was ready to "glide" along the floor from room to room. In this manner I could get around the house somewhat, even though I was now too weak to manage household chores.

On one occasion I managed to get to the kitchen to fix a bowl of soup for Tina who was home with the flu. I had everything on the tray and thought I could manage to carry it to her room, but the pesky cane was in the way and it became impossible. I lost control and ended up on the floor with chicken soup all over my clothes. Tina heard the crash and jumped out of bed to assist me! I am blessed to have children who care!

I couldn't get the 'C' word off my mind. It seemed to haunt me. At the market, the thought of cancer was prevalent. While chatting with my family, I couldn't give them my full attention as cancer was on my mind. When sitting in the pew on Sunday morning, listening to pastor's sermon, the thought of cancer was still with me. No matter where I was or what I was doing, 'cancer'

seemed to override my thoughts. It was difficult to drift into sleep at night as I found myself wondering how I would slip from life on earth to the other side if I should not be a survivor.

Through this trial, I learned what "pray without ceasing" means. I decided that when cancer would be heavy on my mind, I would breathe a prayer for faith and patience. I wondered if I could endure the physical and emotional challenge of the coming days and months. My heart knew without the help of the Lord it would be impossible for me to get through this trial.

Let me share one of the most traumatic events of my life which occurred as a result of chemo. *I awoke one morning to discover my beautiful auburn hair in ringlets on my satin pillow.* Instinctively I ran to the mirror. I was afraid to look, but I had to know. At the sight of my bald head, a gasp escaped my lips. "Ohhhhh noooooo, ohhhhh noooooo I wailed softly to myself in utter horror. I looked like an alien depicted in a TV film. Falling back on the bed, I buried my face in the blankets and sobbed and sobbed. My doctor had told me to expect some hair loss, but I had not expected to lose it all overnight! Again, I was asking, *"What have I done to deserve this?"*

Fortunately Jeff was out of town and the children's rooms were at the other end of the house so they couldn't hear me venting my unhappiness. However they would soon be up preparing for the school day so I had to think fast. What could I do to cover my head? They must never see me like this.

Adrenalin was pumping as I began to look about the room for a solution. I spotted a knit cap in the closet, but that wouldn't do. It was for outdoor wear and would be too obvious at this time of year. Checking my scarf drawer, I found a temporary solution. Selecting a long silk scarf, I began to wind it around my head and tied a bow on top. There wasn't enough bulk, so I had to find something for filler. I located a large piece of half-inch foam from which to fashion a base and rewound the scarf about the foam. This was the best I could do.

The children got up and ate their breakfast without notic-ing a thing! (At least if they did wonder why my head was wrapped in a scarf, they were polite enough not to question me.)   Once Jeremy and Tina had left for school, I scurried around to find a source for head pieces/wigs. A thought occurred: how could I go out into public? There wasn't a wig shop in our little town. What could I do?

Finally I recalled seeing a pamphlet among material given me at the Cancer Center. After a frantic and tiring search, the pamphlet was discovered and I could set a plan in motion.

"Heads Up" is a supplier of specialty wigs made especially for cancer patients. Their offices were only about 70 miles from our home. I called them and was promised a representative would arrive at my home before noon. Their rep, Brenda, arrived at my door all bubbly and excited about helping me select a natural looking wig that would match my basic style and color. She winked at me, asking how I liked her wig?

Soon an array of attractive wigs was set up on the dining room table to make my selection easy. We studied hairstyles and color swatches in order to make the most perfect match. I was beginning to feel a sense of relief. The only catch was that I must wait for at least ten days before delivery. "What will I do in the meantime," I asked Brenda. She was quick to admonish me *not to panic* as she reached into her case for a soft cap of foam rubber which was full of holes for ventilation.

Then Brenda showed me a pretty multi-colored silk head piece that snapped into place over the foam cap. Looking into the mirror, I had to agree it looked quite chic. I would simply adapt a new style until the wig would arrive. When Jeff returned from his sales trip, perhaps I would look halfway decent. Things were looking up.

Two days later Jeff got an early flight and arrived home mid-afternoon. Stepping into the house, he found the children in heated debate over something-or-other. He stepped into the middle of their argument until peace was restored. Then he came to my side to encourage me. He could sense the pressure we were all under due to the changes in our household over the past months. Jeff's presence had a reassuring effect and soon a beautiful feeling of unity filled our home. The children must have felt it too, as they quietly played a board game for the next hour or so.

There was no mention of my new "hairpiece." It seemed my family was totally unaware I had lost my hair. One day while I was chatting on the phone with a friend Jeff took the children aside to explain about my hair loss. To Jeff's amazement Jeremy spoke up brightly, "Oh, we know dad. Mom's really been good about all the changes. She's not making a fuss about it or anything."

My body was experiencing more changes. First, I had lost my hair. Then I began to experience such tremendous weakness after each chemo treatment that lying on the couch, drifting in and out of sleep, became a regular routine. If I was able to get up onto my feet, my wobbly legs didn't want to carry me.

Wretched vomiting began. No matter what I ate, it didn't want to stay down. Food soon lost its savory taste and I wondered why I should even try to eat. It simply wasn't worth the effort. What a bleak existence! Cancer had changed me in ways I truly hated. I became depressed and didn't want to see anyone because I felt deep in my heart nobody would want to see such a wretch as I had become. I especially didn't want my family to see me when dry heaves and/or vomiting took over. A daily shower was replaced with sponge baths as I simply did not have the energy for a shower and a tub bath was out of the question too. I wished for a nurse who could give me bed baths and keep me dressed in clean jammies.

It was difficult to stay fresh and tidy when Jeff was out of town on company business. If Tina was home, I did rely on her from time to time. She could lay out necessities for a sponge bath, including fresh clothes.

> I really miss you when you're gone;
> The hours seem to linger on and on.
> I wait to hear the car turn in the drive
> And listen for your footstep at the door.
> When you step inside and smile as if to say,
> "Honey, I'm home," it's worth the wait,
> Soon your arms wrap 'round me, oh so strong,
> I feel protected and secure once more.

I missed the special times Jeff and I would sit together chatting and interacting with the children. Now I was forced to spend many hours in my room alone, staring at the ceiling and wondering what was going to happen to me.

When my friends came by to clean house they always rapped on my bedroom door to ask what they could do to help me personally. At first it was a delight to have a friend pop in to straighten my room up a bit, plump my pillow and sit for a few moments to visit. However as the disease progressed, I was too ashamed to allow them in the room even though I needed clean sheets and a change of pajamas.

Finally Jeff and I had a talk about the situation and he agreed to start looking for someone who would take complete charge of the house and also take care of my needs. He thanked my friends from the church for their help and informed them their help would no longer be needed as we were in the process of getting a house-keeper.

My sweet children were very brave. If they complained about having to pitch in, I didn't hear it. In retrospect, I know now it was dumb and selfish of me to cancel the team of ladies from our church who were willing to help us. I should have swallowed my pride as Jeff didn't find a housekeeper for quite some time and it put a strain on all of us.

Besides the practical help Jeff could give to the children and me, just having him with us was a joy. He brought laughter and good times into the house. He was always supportive with suggestions and ideas on how to make things better for all of us. I appreciated the fact that he had been able to take me to and from the cancer center on chemo days. Jeff was a most gracious and caring husband. There aren't enough words to express how much his attention to me was appreciated.

When it was necessary for Jeff to travel out of town on business, I missed him tremendously. However our marriage was strong. He kept in touch by calling at least twice a day. In the event of an emergency, I only needed to press a special button on a chain around my neck and be in touch with 911.

Jeff's company was in the process of negotiating a merger which often required his attendance at evening meetings. I understood as an officer of the firm he must work late in planning meetings. With his experience and knowledge, plus his unique ability to make presentations, he was the preferred traveler to Atlanta, Denver or wherever they needed representation.

However, Jeremy and Tina were not patient. They felt their dad should be home helping us. Often I heard them pleading with their father, "Please don't be late tonight." It hurt to know they were alone when I was a prisoner in my room who wanted desperately to continue to be a sweet, caring mother while daddy was away on business.

No doubt about it, *people do need people* contact. After a month or so of hiding away I was gripped with an overwhelming feeling of loneliness and realized I needed contact with my old friends. I began calling some of them, only to discover there were few pleasantries I could think of which might interest them. Surely they had little interest in hearing details of my dismal existence, so I stopped calling and did not encourage them to call me. It was also discouraging to hear their animated conversation as they related to me the exciting events occurring in their households.

I absolutely had to get well in order to enjoy again the wonderful times our family had together. It would be a great day when I could return to my role as companion to my husband and children.

✝✝✝

A wonderful surprise greeted me one day when I answered the doorbell. Two of my college roommates from the University of Oregon embraced me. We spent the afternoon recalling fun college days. They made stimulating conversation and it felt *awfully good* to laugh again.

After awhile Marge excused herself to visit the bathroom. Katie began asking a lot of questions about my treatment, etc., but I was interested in hearing about *her* family and what *they* were doing. Actually Marge was in the kitchen cleaning up the clutter. When she finished, everything was sparkling. I can't thank her enough for her generous gesture.

Marge asked if I had considered getting a housekeeper. I told her ladies from the church had come to clean one day a week until Jeff told them we were in the process of getting a housekeeper. Marge told me it was foolish to deprive my family of needed assistance and I knew she was right. Was I suffering from false pride?

Somewhat reluctantly I said goodbye to my friends. They were both in excellent health, had married well and knew the joy of children. Watching them from the open doorway, it wasn't easy to keep from feeling jealous of my dear friends. They enjoyed an active life. If I were perfectly honest, I'd have to admit twinges of remorse over my physical situation. These gals still had half of their lives ahead of them. They looked forward to a bright future each day.

I shuffled to the bedroom where I picked up the Bible to encourage myself. I was on the teeter-totter again! Too many changes were happening and I wasn't prepared for them. In the past, I had always been involved in social activities among my circle of friends. Now I was out of the loop and I didn't like it. I knew then I must get well in order to have friends over occasionally for a special dinner or barbecue in the nearby park.

Do you sometimes feel alone, when you need someone to talk to?

Do you sometimes feel alone when you'd like to just sit and listen to a friend and laugh?

Being alone could turn into a blessing as it gives one the opportunity to pick up a magazine or a good book you haven't finished.

Here's another idea - have you thought of keeping a journal? Your day's activities may someday be of interest to you once you've received news you're free of cancer. You may smile at yourself while reading some entries or cry at other comments you penned while battling debilitating disease.

A journal may also be of interest to family members at some point. Just think, thoughts you put in the journal may become an interesting part of history.

You won't feel so alone if you can do something to create an interesting day-to-day existence for yourself. As long as you have energy, find ways to keep your mind busy. Work on any hobbies such as writing or scrapbooking, cataloging photos, etc., as long as you can.

INSPIRATION

"He giveth power to the faint and to them
that have no might He increaseth strength."
Isaiah 40:29

APPLICATION

Praise the Lord for His goodness. I gave my heart
to the Lord at the age of 14 and have never cared to
try the sins of the world. Memories are pleasant.
There are no regrets.

Through the affliction of a disease where there has
only been minimal research, I have learned to fully
trust in Jesus. I lean hard upon His word for it gives
me HOPE and PEACE. The Word gives me POW-
ER to fight harder against the ravages of disease.
The Word gives me JOY in place of sadness and
despair.

I pray to retain this joy and peace. "Thank you, Lord
for the strength I have derived from your living Word.
Help me hold onto your truth and not be overcome
with fear of the unknown tomorrow."

COME UNTO ME ALL YOU WHO LABOR AND ARE HEAVY LADEN, AND I WILL GIVE YOU REST.

MATTHEW 11:28

3

What have I Done to Deserve This?

When Dr. Nelson initially gave me the news of cancer, I had no idea confinement in the house would become routine. My gardening days had long ago come to an abrupt halt. We had 42 different varieties of prize winning fragrant roses in the garden that needed ongoing attention.

I called a neighbor to get the name of her gardener. Having arranged for him to begin work on our garden, I felt a deep sense of relief, knowing our property would soon be in A-1 shape again. To top it off, we would soon have vases of lovely flowers bringing sweet per-fume into our home.

For whatever reason I felt I needed to make a tour of the house, something I hadn't done in a few weeks. With the aid of my cane I shuffled carefully from room to room. The bathroom shared by the children looked as pitiful as the rose garden. There were no pretty towels on the rods. Instead they had been thrown in haste on-to the floor. The children's clothes were scattered about. I bent down to pick them up, but soon realized it was a mistake as I tripped and almost fell.

Stepping into Tina's room, it was plain to see the floor had not been vacuumed in some time. Activity books, dolls and doll clothes were in disarray on the floor. I couldn't help but wonder when the bed sheets had been changed last. With some effort, I managed to walk around the bed and pull the sheets off. My energy was expended in Tina's room so I decided Jeremy could remove the sheets from his bed.

Thinking I could wash a load of bedding, I dragged the soiled sheets behind me to the laundry room. One of my scuffs became tangled in the bedding and I lost my footing. My cane swung upward, striking me in the forearm and I fell to the floor. For a few moments, I lay there, dazed and embarrassed even though there was nobody to see me splat-out on the floor.

Soon I was in tears again. I didn't have the strength to call out, and no one would hear me if I could. I lay in a heap of laundry whimpering, "Why can't I get well? I can't take it anymore." I felt too foolish to press the button that would bring help.

My world was falling apart. As a wife and mother, it was my job (and privilege) to keep the household chores done but cancer had reduced me to staying in bed much of the time. It was discouraging to note the neglect throughout our lovely home and not be able to do anything about it.

While all this was going on Jeff had been trying to call me. As I wasn't answering the phone, he sensed something must be wrong and raced home to check on me. I had heard the phone ringing, but was tangled up in the bedding and knew I could never get to it in time so it went unanswered. Jeff arrived and rushed into the house. He was calling my name as he ran from room to room.   He was surprised to discover me in a heap of soiled linens on the laundry room floor. When he saw I had been weeping he picked me up and carried me to the big soft chaise lounge in the family room.

Jeff poured a glass of cold, icy lemonade for both of us and we began to discuss the situation at hand.   He scolded me for trying to do laundry. I pleaded with him that I had to put some effort into making things better for the family.

I knew in my heart we had to have help with household chores if the children were to grow up in an orderly home. It didn't seem fair to burden 10- and 12-year-old Tina and Jeremy with housework when they had school activities, athletic games and music lessons besides their schoolwork. And Jeff had obligations with his company that required him to work late at the office many evenings, besides somewhat frequent out-of-town business trips.

My family deserved better than this, but I was limited in what I could contribute. "Jeff, I want to work in the flowers, but I cannot. I want to walk down to the lake, but I cannot. I want to do the laundry and bake a cake and keep the house tidy as I used to do, but I cannot. What are we going to do?"

Jeff was sitting on the hearth just looking at me. I'm sure he didn't know what to say. Finally I broke the ice by asking him if he thought I would ever get better. "I certainly am looking forward to it, Hon," was his quick reply, but not with a lot of conviction. I began to press Jeff about his most recent discussion with Dr. Unruh. Jeff told me he felt the doctor was somewhat evasive, as he hadn't given him a direct answer. However, the doctor admitted the chemo wasn't working as he had hoped.

Hearing these words sent a chill down my back and my eyes became misty. I felt I was sinking and would sure-ly drown. Sometimes I cried until my eyes were dry. Before the onset of cancer I felt invincible. I was young. I was strong; I had a super good husband and the best two kids in the world. We were the ideal family with all we could hope for and now I have a terminal disease!

Through this traumatic turn of events I discovered my emotions were as thin as tissue paper. Thankfully, Jeff was strong. When I was about to sink into deep water, he would come along and lift my spirits. At other times this caring sweetness would reach out to me from a perfect stranger. Once I was sitting alone in a hospital chapel, crying softly when a stranger touched me on the shoulder and told me to "trust in God and everything will come out alright."

Jeff spoke up, bringing me back to the present. He suggested it was a good time to take a little drive up the coast. The children wouldn't be home from school for several hours and it would be great to have a change of scenery. He helped me into the car which was a feat in itself. Driving north, we were soon in the town of Bandon. Jeff found a place to stop where it seemed we could see forever. Oh how I loved the breathtaking beauty of the Pacific coastline.

We sat on a park bench with the warm sun on our backs. Soon our pressing problems receded to the background as we relaxed to the gentle surf playing along the sandy shore. It was good to get out of the depressing house for a short time. Jeff needed it as much as I. It must have been difficult for him to watch me waste away a day at a time and he couldn't stop it.

Dr. Unruh announced it was time to become more aggressive with the treatment. I had to remain close to my bathroom as the wretched vomiting attacked with a vengeance. If my stomach was empty, dry heaves took over – what an unpleasant event!

I tried to spend as much time as possible with my family. If I didn't feel like participating in a board game or working a puzzle, I could at least be in the room with them. I put a lot of effort into keeping an upbeat personality regardless of how I may have been feeling. It was important for the children to have a measure of normalcy in our home.

However, socializing with the children came to an abrupt halt when the disease picked up pace. Leaving my room became a rarity. In the past, one of the things I enjoyed most was the time spent with my children. Brushing Tina's hair had been a daily event. She would be bubbling over about friends, school and whatever may have happened that day. I had continued to brush her hair until I lost strength in my arms. Jeremy had taken an interest in ironing his own shirts so I coached him in the proper method. Most of his clothing was wrinkle-free so his ironing was minimal.

Jeff knew how long the days were for me. He apologized frequently when he had to travel on business. He also knew music had been a big part of my life. He purchased a mix of new gospel and classical DVD's and placed them on the nightstand next to the portable DVD player. This wonderful music would feed my soul, making each day a little more bearable.

A particular chorus that lifted my spirits from one day to the next was: *"Someone to care; someone to share all your troubles like no other can do. He'll come down from the skies and brush the tears from your eyes. You're His child and He cares for you!"* (author unknown.) If I were able to sing along, I'd substitute "my" for "your" to personalize the tremendous thought that there was someone who cared for me. It was truly awesome to realize that Jesus was interceding for me. What more could I hope for?

The disease affected my mental state so I couldn't be upbeat all the time. As mentioned before, I kept getting onto the teeter-totter. I'd be up one day and down the next. It was amazing how Jeremy and Tina put up with my mood swings. Maybe their dad told them to expect personality changes. I never wanted to withdraw from them, but when days were filled with wretched vomiting and dry heaves I had to remain in my room.

Caregivers, persons who are terminally ill need quiet time to themselves, but it's also important for them to be included in family activities even though they may only be a spectator.

There is a certain amount of care that must be given by others when one is too ill to handle his or her own personal needs. This thought applies to the spiritual well-being as well as the physical. We who are ill need daily encouragement. It's true that through the pressure of adversity we are molded more and more in Christ's image - that is, if we keep a sweet spirit and do not allow our-selves to be swallowed up in bitterness.

Surely you want to be known as a sweet person of courage and faith in troubled times If life dishes out a plate of trial and disappointment, that's the time to trust in God with all that is within you. If you ask Him, He will give you a measure of peace equal to your need.

I was no different from millions of others with terminal disease who don't understand why bad things happen to good people. We obeyed the rules we think are necessary to obtain a normal life free of hardship.

Many hours passed while I tried in my finite mind to discover why I had been afflicted with a life-threatening disease. Cancer may be hereditary or the result of a lifestyle we have chosen or a direct result of having been exposed to carcinogens in some way.

When we suffer, why are we so quick to think God is punishing us? We are His children and He does want good things for us. Perhaps we can stop trying to discover "WHY" (for we may never attain the answer we want) and live one day at a time.

Many months had passed since I heard the 'C' word which changed my world. I had now overcome the initial trauma and should have been thinking with clarity. It has been said that a patient who maintains a positive attitude in spite of the disease is much more likely to recover than one who goes to bed and pulls the covers up over his/her head.

Again I struggled against self-pity, partially due to lonely days and nights when I longed for someone to sit beside my bed quietly visiting or reading the Bible to bring cheer into my day. It was evident chemo wasn't doing its job and I wondered if there would be a 'tomorrow' for me. I had no quality of life and was beginning to feel I would not win this battle and I desperately wanted to live. I could only see dark days ahead and wondered where all the sunny days had gone.

I didn't want to be on the teeter-totter again, so I decided to concentrate on HOPE. I needed to keep from being discouraged and feeling such a deep sense of loss. I knew in my heart if I could live one day at a time and not think of tomorrow, I could survive. I determined to live for NOW. There was so much to live for: family and good friends who care about me. I shall try to turn my sadness into uplifting HOPE.

For many years I thought I was trusting God to provide for each day. Now I realize I have a tendency to keep picking my burdens back up, so I am working on becoming stronger in the Word in order to abandon my cares completely to Jesus who is watching over me every hour of the day and night.

When I saturated myself with inspiration that comes from above, I was stronger emotionally. I was in a mode of remembering passages of scripture I had known for many years. Now it was time to share these positive and encouraging thoughts with family and friends. They needed to feel a sense of encouragement not only *for* me, but also *from* me.

I learned to avoid people who stand in the shadows whispering such thoughts as, "What a shame...and she's so young to die - so sad for the children what will they do without a mother - how will they manage when their father travels out of town, etc."

Reader, you, must close your ears to careless comments that lack consideration for your feelings. It's easy, though certainly not wise to speak without thinking. Learn to turn aside from discouraging comments. You don't need to hear them. Distance yourself from persons who seem to be full of discouraging words. As much as you can, surround yourself with beautiful things such as family photos, remembering happy times on vacations, picnics, birthdays and/or other celebrations.

People are often too quick to speak without thinking. We have all done it from time to time. It's most important for you to close your ears to discouraging statements. You don't need to hear them.

Listen to scripture tapes, CD's, inspirational music or relaxing music of nature. Perhaps your family can set up a 'music center' at your bedside. Music that lifts up the Lord, giving Him praise, is healing to the soul and good for your emotional and physical well being.

Here I am Again Lord

Here I am again Lord; I've been reading in Your Word and claiming promises for answered prayer.

> "Is any sick among you? Let him call for the elders of the church; and let them pray over him, anointing him with oil in the name of the Lord: and the prayer of faith shall save the sick and the Lord shall raise him up; and if he has committed sins they shall be forgiven him." James 5:13,14

I do not know how long I shall live. My thoughts and prayers arise to God who created me, asking that the cancerous cells that have invaded my body would shrivel and die. It is my greatest desire to live, to do something worthy, to be a blessing to others who may cross my path from day to day.

I have been praying and the church has also prayed for my healing but I am not getting better. Perhaps I should consider a fact to be reckoned with: my *days are numbered*. When it is time for me to go to my eternal reward, I shall fly away to Glory!

4

Helping Others

The morning sun and fresh sea air beckoned me outdoors. With some effort, I shuffled through the house to
the patio, my favorite place. The school bus had picked
up Jeremy and Tina; I was sipping my English breakfast
tea in quiet solitude. I had been free of wretched vomiting for a day or so.

Cat was curled up at my feet. "How I love this place," I
thought. The gardener was keeping our rose garden in
tip-top shape. Their fragrant blooms were delightful.
The water very gently played along the lakeshore. It was
a quiet, perfect beginning of a brand new day.

Soon I heard the telephone ringing. I wasn't very frisky anymore and consequently made no effort to get to the phone. Let it ring. The caller could leave a message. Later, when I took the call, I was surprised to hear my friend, Tex. She sounded troubled and asked me to call her.

Dialing Tex's number, I couldn't imagine what her problem could be. It seemed everything always went her way. She had a beautiful life, never interrupted by a negative. There were no ripples to bother her, or so it seemed. Tex answered my call and said she needed to talk. Could she come right over? I invited her over and in 20 minutes she was sitting with me on the patio.

Tex seemed somewhat reticent to talk about what was troubling her. She finally blurted out, "My doctor found a lump in my breast!" Her chin quivered as tears spilled from her eyes. I knew exactly how frightened she was and began searching for comforting words I could say that might diminish the blow of the 'C' word.

Reaching across the patio table, I took her hand in mine. "Oh Tex, I know exactly how you feel. When did you find out," I asked her. Tex was dabbing at her eyes with a tissue. Looking up, she explained she had known for two days and couldn't believe it was true. She wanted to know if I had the same feelings when I first heard the 'C' word. I assured her it's a natural human response to go into denial as cancer is the last thing one would ever wish to deal with.

As friends do, we spent a good deal of time comparing our feelings and trying to determine how best to deal with this new knowledge. We both felt afraid, anxious and fearful of the unknown.

A cool breeze began to blow over the water and it was suggested we move into the house where it would be more comfortable. Once we were seated in the den, I reached for the Bible to give a word of hope and encouragement to my close friend. The Word would equip her to better face this new trial.

I encouraged Tex to trust in the Lord as His promises are forever. They will never fail if we believe. When we cannot trust in ourselves, our family or the doctor, we can always trust in the Lord. His word is truth. Millions upon millions of people all over the world put their faith in Jesus every day.

Tex admitted to loving the Lord and striving to do His will. She had been a Christian for eight years. However, she was possessed with a fear that her husband would no longer love her after the mastectomy. "What!" I exclaimed, "Teddy will love you just the same." Tex jumped up and began walking nervously around the room. Stopping directly in front of me, she asserted, "But I'll be...I'll be mutilated! My breast will be gone!"

I assured Tex that Teddy loved her for who she was and surgery would make no difference in his lifelong commitment of marriage. He would be beside her all the way. Also, she could lean on me when she felt alone.

"Know therefore that the Lord thy God,
He *is* God, the *faithful* God, which keepeth
covenant and mercy with them that love
Him and keep His commandments
to a thousand generations."
Deut. 7:9 KJV

To encourage ourselves, Tex and I began to reiterate the many events of healing and answered prayer in our local church. We remembered Aunt Fannie who was healed of crippling arthritis after many years of suffering.

She hadn't been able to play the piano for over ten years due to arthritic pain in her hands. After healing, her music ministry was renewed. Then there was four-year-old Bobby Garvey who was healed of leukemia when doctors said there was nothing else they could do for him. Now, at the age of seven, this active child had no apparent physical, emotional or mental problems because of the steadfast prayers of our church.

As Christians, we both knew God could do anything if we only believed. There was no doubt in our minds but that we would both be healed. Our faith began to lift until we were walking on cloud nine when Tex stood up to go. I prayed for Tex and encouraged her not to *panic.* To panic indicates we see absolutely no way out. If we are trusting in the Lord, we *do* see a way out, for we *know* without a shadow of doubt that He *will* provide a way.

> Reader the direction *our Lord chooses for us may not always be the path we would choose, but we continue to trust Him just the same. He knows all things and has a particular plan for our lives.*

I urged Tex to keep in touch. When she left I felt elated, elevated and excited that in spite of my infirmity I had been able to encourage her and hopefully lift her faith. My friend had departed and I knelt to thank the Lord for sending Tex to me. I wanted to be a source of blessing to others. Perhaps the Lord could send hurting and needy people to my doorstep. If I could not go where they were, He might put them in my path.

Through this experience I learned a valuable lesson: *one must not back out of life because he/she is ill.* It is no excuse for overlooking the needs of others around us. I had a new realization of purpose in my life. I could be an instrument of encouragement even while I, myself, was struggling for victory.

Also, I was reminded that I was not alone in suffering. It seemed that more and more people were being diagnosed with cancer. Folk all around me were reaching out for someone to help them, someone to care, someone to share the burden. Many of them were finding solace and comfort through their church and the local pastor. We were hearing of other cancer patients who were being healed and going into remission.

Tex and I did keep in touch. The next week she called me about a wonderful experience she had while in the hospital. Her doctor was consulting with another surgeon in the hallway while Tex lay on the hospital bed. She could hear little snatches of conversation and, fearing the worst, began to weep softly. Things were happening too fast! She felt a sense of panic when suddenly it seemed she heard the voice of the Lord gently whisper, "I am taking care of you." Immediately she could relax with the profound knowledge she was in her heavenly Father's care.

Tex went into the operating room with renewed peace that everything was going to be alright. She had the surgery and a schedule for chemotherapy was established. Interestingly enough, the chemo did not have the same effect on Tex as it had on me.

Each session drained her of some energy, but after a day or two she was able to resume her normal activities. Best of all, her appetite was good and she did not experience any bouts of vomiting. After three months of chemo, Tex noticed her hair was thinning slightly, but it never fell out completely as mine had. I was happy for my friend.

We chatted frequently on the telephone and Tex kept encouraging me that I would soon turn a curve in the road and the cancer would go into remission. I don't know what I'd have done without my friend's encouragement. She knew exactly what I was going through.

Once it became an effort to get dressed for church on Sunday, I began to stay home. The services were too long for me to endure sitting in the hard pew. Besides, many of my old friends now seemed somewhat distant, as though they feared they might *catch* cancer from me. I didn't want their pity; I only hoped for their continued friendship and support during this difficult time. In the past, I was in the inner circle where I knew everything that was happening. Now I was excluded – on the outside. Since my illness, I had given it a great deal of thought.

It occurred to me that we must have appeared as snobs to others who may have felt as I do now, ostracized and shut out. Now that I was on the 'outside,' I saw more clearly and asked the Lord to forgive me for my former snobbish behavior.

So here I was alone on another Sunday morning when I'd much rather have been in church. Jeff had made me comfortable in the family room so that I could enjoy a Christian TV program. I was halfway reclining in my chair when the doorbell rang. It wasn't going to be easy to get the door. I was wondering who would be calling on a Sunday morning. I called out, "Just a minute," while slipping out of the recliner and into my scuffs.

What a surprise to find my neighbor, Mrs. Rankin, at the door. She said she noticed I had not gone to church with the family and had come over to keep me company. I thanked her for the gesture and invited her in.

It wasn't long until Mrs. Rankin began to tell me about a pressing problem in their home. It seemed her husband wasn't coming directly home from work anymore. He was paying less and less attention to her and slipping away to another room out of her hearing having hushed conversations with someone on his cell phone. She had concluded her husband must be talking with another woman. However, when she recently confronted him about his clandestine conversations, he denied any friendship with another woman.

Mrs. Rankin wanted advice: what should she do? She felt cut off from her husband and was certain he was having an affair with another woman. This was a difficult question to answer. I knew nothing of the matter. "I'm sorry you are going through this difficult time," I told her, "but we really don't know what is going on with your husband do we?" She was quick to agree. As we talked further, she came to the realization perhaps she should believe her husband was telling the truth when he said there was 'no other woman.'

I had made a habit of reading the Bible and watching electronic church during the time my family would be attending services in town. I asked my neighbor if she would like to join me in Bible reading and, after some hesitation, she agreed to it. A Christian TV program was still on. Though I had earlier turned the volume down, I now turned the TV off in order to concentrate on discussion with my neighbor. My mind was racing, trying to think of appropriate scripture that would be helpful to Mrs. Rankin. This time together with my neighbor would hopefully turn out to be a blessing to her.

I had no idea what her spiritual life was, however I felt a strong urge to read a salvation passage. Turning to the third chapter of John, (in the New Testament), I began to read a key verse from the Bible:

> *"For God so loved the world that He gave His only begotten son that whosoever believeth in Him should not perish but have eternal life."*
> John 3:16

It was evident to me God had brought my neighbor to me for a reason. I had to discover if she knew the Lord as her personal Savior. Going back and repeating verses 15, 16 and 17, I elaborated on the gift of eternal life and that Jesus had not come into the world to condemn the world, but to forgive our sins and give us eternal life.

My neighbor smiled broadly while exclaiming she felt a heavy load had lifted from her. Soon she began to tell me she had once known the Lord, but had drifted into the world when she got married 21 years ago. I had been asking the Lord to make me a blessing to others, and now I had a wonderful opportunity to help my neighbor. It was exhilarating - my spirits were lifted.

I prayed with her, leading her back into fellowship with the Lord. She began to pray, asking the Lord to forgive her sins and give her peace again. We had prayed together for her husband and put him in the hands of the Lord.

When Mrs. Rankin walked back into her house she carried several Christian magazines which she dropped on the coffee table. Her husband, who was watching the sports channel on TV, asked her where she had been and he wanted to know what kind of magazines she had.

This gave her a good opportunity to tell him she had just rededicated her life to the Lord. "The car's still here so it's obvious you haven't been to church. How did you do that rededication thing you're talking about," he asked. Mrs. Rankin explained she had gone next door to keep her sick neighbor company while her family had gone to church. She told him their neighbor, in spite of her illness, had taken the time to talk with her about the love of God and salvation.

Mr. Rankin could see new light in his wife's eyes and she was all bubbly and excited. All he could manage to say was, "Good deal." After a few minutes he seemed restless and left the room.

Mrs. Rankin began making Sunday dinner while her husband stood looking out the window that faced our property. He had decided perhaps he should visit Jeff who might be able to help him through a crucial situation he was going through. He was waiting for Jeff to return home from church. Finally, when he saw Jeff's car enter our property, he left by the back door and crossed quickly into our yard where he knocked on the kitchen door.

As my family had barely come into the house, I had not yet had a chance to share the excitement about Mrs. Rankin's visit before her husband was being invited in by Jeff. Mr. Rankin seemed somewhat nervous for a moment; then he asked if Jeff had a few minutes to talk privately. He knew Jeff was a Christian man and he needed someone to confide in over a serious personal matter.

Jeff took Mr. Rankin into the family room where they could talk undisturbed while I situated the children at the kitchen table. Under my supervision, Jeremy and Tina took vegetables from the refrigerator to prepare a salad. While sitting at the table, I was able to slice cheese and apply mayonnaise to slices of bread. Ham and cheese was put on the bread along with lettuce. Now we were ready for lunch whenever Jeff and our neighbor would finish their discussion.

While the children and I prepared lunch our neighbor was asking Jeff for serious advice. It seems he had become involved in some sort of money-making-scheme-gone-bad. He wanted to get out of the organization, but was afraid of reprisals.

When Jeff asked him if he knew the Lord, Mr. Rankin admitted to having gone to Sunday School as a child. He said he had drifted far into the world and wasn't sure if God would have anything to do with him. Jeff assured him of God's forgiveness as he quoted John 3:16. (What a coincidence that both of us used the same salvation scripture in witnessing to our friends.) He reminded Mr. Rankin of God's forgiving love that had placed Jesus on the cross to bear our sins. "Would you let me pray with you," Jeff asked our neighbor. (Prayer was natural for our family. We prayed about many things, always prior to making a critical decision.) Mr. Rankin agreed and soon was confessing his sins and asking the Lord for forgiveness. He rededicated his life to Christ. Jeff prayed for Him and the critical situation that confronted him.

Jeff promised to introduce our neighbor to someone on the following day that might possibly be able to assist Mr. Rankin in the delicate situation he was in.

While Mr. Rankin was talking and praying with Jeff, his wife observed he was no longer in their house. Frantically, she called our home to announce he had disappeared and she suspected some kind of foul play. Would I pray? She was surprised to learn her husband was in our home and quickly ran from her house and arrived, breathless, at our front door. It was wonderful to see the Rankins embrace and share the excitement of their new commitments to the Lord. Surely the Lord works in marvelous ways!

From time to time there were other people the Lord put in my path for spiritual help. More and more *I came to realize my infirmity had become an opportunity for ministry.* Now on my chemo days I became cognizant of other cancer patients in the waiting room. I was able to speak a word of encouragement to them as we had a common goal: fighting cancer.

On one visit to the medical office I had just gotten settled in the waiting room when I saw a figure resting on the floor. As I gazed upon her, she lifted her head and our eyes met. Her skin was deeply wrinkled and leathery looking as though she may have been a sun worshiper through the years. Her eyes were deeply set in a misshapen face. There was a look of fear and apprehension about her.

Judging by her appearance, I felt she undoubtedly had little means of income. I was drawn to her, but didn't feel at ease to begin a conversation in the crowded waiting room.

Later as I was leaving the facility I noticed this woman standing outside the entry doors. "I saw you inside," I began. "How are you today?" She seemed surprised that I noticed her. "How do you think I am? I've got cancer same as you," was her somewhat gruff reply. "I know. It's not fun for any of us," I continued. Instantly she grabbed onto my arm and looked directly into my face. "Do you got somebody to help you," she blurted out. "I don't got nobody, I'm all alone. I suffer alone. I'll die alone. There ain't nobody to care about Sarah," she remarked bitterly.

My heart went out to my new friend. "Why Sarah, I care. Let me be your friend." I reached into my bag to retrieve a small notepad so that I could get Sarah's address and phone number.

At that moment Jeff drove up to the curb. Stepping to the car as he rolled the window down, I mentioned my new friend and that I had offered to take her home. Though she was waiting for a bus, taking her home would allow an opportunity to get acquainted. I held the door open and somewhat timidly she did get into the back seat. Almost instantly she blurted out, "Boy oh boy, I ain't nevah rode in such a fancy car. I shoulda took the bus like I said." Jeff was quick to respond with, "Sarah, It's our pleasure to take you home."

We arrived at Sarah's tiny unassuming house. The appearance suggested it had been erected many years ago. In need of paint, it sat on a dreary lot littered with old mattresses and car parts long ago discarded. The windows were only partially covered by tattered cloth that at one time may have been pretty curtains. We pretended not to notice. Jeff opened the car door for her and I got out too. Reaching for her hand, I promised to check in on her from time to time. She turned toward her house, then quickly spun around and grabbed me by the shoulder. "You're the first folk to ever notice Sarah. You've been kind. I'll not forget you," she blurted out. And then Jeff and I were on our way. It felt good to lift a tiny bit of the burden Sarah carries.

I Talked with God

I talked with God today; I heard Him call my name.
I talked with God today; I'll never be the same.
I talked with God today and remembered you there.
I talked with God today when I knelt in prayer.
I told Him everything – how I cared about you.
Now in my heart I sing; His word is true.
I talked with God today, I heard Him say,
"My child, the answer's on the way."

One Sunday night Jeff returned from church and mentioned Tex was there and had asked for special prayer.

Though she had the surgery and had been on chemo for some time, her recent 'cancer count' was higher than it should have been. I knew how important the cancer count was and my heart went out to her. I also knew exactly how she must be feeling and I sincerely prayed she would be healed.

Reader, when doctors say there is no hope, or you receive a negative report, keep trusting the Lord. You don't know what the future holds, but you are secure in Him for whatever may develop today, tomorrow and the next day!

There is an element of mystery in knowing God's will. He knows some of us would drive our car off a cliff if we knew the future, so in His magnificent love, He shields us from this knowledge.

Tex called to let me know she would be seeing her doctor again in a few days. She mentioned the special prayer on her behalf the previous Sunday night and said she actually had been feeling quite a lot better.

Friday arrived and Tex asked her doctor to order new lab work to determine if perhaps her cancer count was down now. With some reluctance her doctor agreed if she were still feeling better in two weeks, he would order a new lab. Praise the Lord, new lab work indicated the cancer count *was* down and Tex was elated!

Chemo continued. A few months later Tex received the good news that *cancer was in remission.* She had to share the good news. She called our pastor and many friends to share the answer to prayer. We rejoiced together. Pastor Murphy was not at all surprised at the good report. Hadn't they prayed for healing? Only Tex's doctor was perplexed as he had not counted on a quick recovery for his patient. Tex knew in her heart the Lord had performed a miracle in answer to prayer.

Tex wanted to give something back to the Lord for her healing. She made contact with a cancer center and began a visitation ministry to other patients who needed a little cheering up. She read cards and letters from their loved ones and became a new friend.

My faith was rising. I could have the same good results as my friend, Tex. I had prayed for healing and the church had prayed for me. Surely there aren't any favorites with God.

Friend, God does *not* have favorites. For reasons unknown to us, all prayers are not answered in the exact way we would prefer. It appears that God, in his infinite wisdom often chooses to take one of His children home where they will instantly be healed of all disease – beautiful again! There will be no more pain, grief or anguish in Heaven. Praise God for His enduring love!

Inspiration

"Delight thyself also in the Lord and He shall give thee the desires of thine heart." Psalm 37:4

Application

I am delighting myself in the Lord. Since the diagnosis of cancer during the past year I have trusted in the Word more than ever. I have put scripture promises where I see them every day to be reminded of God's faithfulness to me.

I continue to hold the thought one day soon I shall be well again – energetic and active. If I can stay off the teeter-totter and be more emotionally stable, the long days and nights will go by more quickly.

The desire of my heart is to know cancer has been eradicated from my frail body and a healthy appetite will be restored. To again savor the taste of good food will be a most pleasant experience. It will be pure joy to gain back some of the weight lost through this struggle. "Oh, Lord, please give me the desires of my heart."

5

Chemotherapy Fails

My life had become pretty bleak since chemo began. Stubborn cancer was not responding as hoped. After a few months of chemo I could no longer go out socially. Much of the time I was alone in my home while Jeff was at work and the children were in school.

One day turned into another with little excitement. However, I looked forward to Saturday mornings when my sister would call. Her purpose was to cheer me and plant a seed of faith in my heart – and it worked. New hope always lifted my spirits.

My sister was always upbeat. She and her husband seemed to have faith that moved mountains. She had personally experienced many answers to her prayer needs and kept reminding me that *nothing is impossible with God*. She would read portions of scripture and pray with me over the telephone, which greatly encouraged me and gave me strength to face another day.

Dr. Unruh checked my cancer count periodically to determine if the chemo was having the desired effect on the disease. If recent lab work indicated the cancer number was down, my sister would rejoice with me. If the cancer count was up, she would give me a new promise from the Word and pray about it with me. Her calls were like a long distance pastoral visit for they encouraged me and helped me face another day.

I awoke today feeling more energetic than usual. I grabbed my trusty cane and glided along the floor in my scuffs to the kitchen where Jeremy and Tina were making instant flavored oatmeal in the microwave. I sipped a cup of tea and ate a few bites of oatmeal with my two special people. All too soon the bus arrived and they kissed me on the cheek and ran out of the house. To my surprise, the oatmeal stayed down. I would have to try it more often.

Glancing out the kitchen window, I enjoyed the sight of our rose garden. There hadn't been a vase of flowers in the house for some time. Perhaps I could go out and cut a few fragrant blooms.

As I was pondering whether to go outdoors, Jeff called from Denver where he had been in meetings for the past two days. Aware of my frail make-up at this time, he encouraged me not to venture into the garden alone. If I could wait until the next day, he would be home in the early afternoon and then we could spend some time together in the garden.

How could I not go to my garden when the bright sun beckoned me outdoors! Puffy Oregon clouds drifted along in the sunshine overhead. Like a naughty child, I paid no attention to Jeff and, with shears in hand, began to cut blooms from our roses. It felt so good to be out-doors and soon I was humming a Mosie Lister tune: *"Oh, I woke up this mornin' feeling fine; I woke up with heav'n on my mind. I woke up with joy in my soul, for I knew that my Lord had control..."* These words expressed how I truly felt at the moment. The air was just a little nippy out, but pleasant. It had been a long time since I'd been outdoors and I savored every moment.

Jeff and I knew most of our roses by name. I pressed my nose into "Medallion," a huge delicate peach-colored rose with a most marvelous fragrance. I was unaware of a wasp among the fragrant petals until the insect began buzzing around my head. It frightened me. Not sure what to do, I froze. The bee, less timid, stung me on the neck with vengeance.

At that point, my immediate reaction was to start squealing and going in circles. Mrs. Rankin, who was standing at her mailbox, could see something unusual was happening and ran across the lot to see what the problem was.

She led me to a bench on the patio and I pointed to my neck where the stinger had been embedded by the wasp. Mrs. Rankin ran back to her house to retrieve a pair of tweezers in order to remove the stinger. She had barely left my side when another wasp buzzed by. I grabbed my cane and headed for the house, because I didn't want to be stung again. In my haste, I tripped over a loose brick in the patio floor and fell.

Jeff was right. I wasn't strong enough to be standing in the garden cutting flowers. I should have followed his advice and stayed indoors until he returned. Soon my neighbor returned, surprised to find me sprawled out on the brick patio. Once the stinger was removed she led me into the house where she applied an old fashioned poultice of soda to draw out the poison. Mrs. Rankin made me comfortable on the couch in the family room before returning to her home.

When Tina came in from school she discovered me asleep on the couch. My neck was swollen and red. Knowing it could be serious, Tina began calling, "Mom, wake up. Something's wrong with your neck." She brought a mirror and I could see the result of the bee sting. When I explained to Tina about the wasp, she immediately went to the phone and dialed 911. Within minutes the house was full of paramedics, firemen and even a policeman. Genuine concern was evident as the paramedics were on-line with the hospital emergency room getting specific instructions for treatment. Once their job was done the house was quiet again.

I fell asleep for a short nap and awakened to discover Tina sleeping, curled up in a chair with Cat in her lap. It had been a long and exciting day for her too. I sat watching her for a few moments, thankful and pleased that she had known how to handle the bee sting crisis. Tina was quite grown up for a 10-year-old. I looked upon her face and felt a twinge of pain. She's pretty and so blessed with grace. Looking at her I knew deep in my heart there was a strong possibility I might soon be going away and leaving my dear daughter. Will she grow up to be like me, even though I may not be there to shape her future?

I reached for my Bible and found this promise that was appropriate for me: "*In the time of trouble He shall hide me in His pavilion; in the secret of His tabernacle shall He hide me. He shall set me up upon a rock.*" Psalm 27:5 What a blessing this verse was! I read it over and over again to absorb the full meaning. Cancer certainly was making me more dependent on others.

However I knew if Jesus set me upon a rock, as the Word declared, I was safe. Chilly water might be pounding forcefully against the rock, but if I would cling to it in the name of the Lord He would pluck me away to safety. The key is to hold fast and wait for His timely deliverance.

When Tina awoke, she chided me for working in the garden and made me promise I wouldn't do it again unless someone was with me. I didn't tell her I had fallen, but later in the evening the Rankins came by to check on me and they mentioned the fall.

The following afternoon Jeff flew back home. It was impossible to keep my journey into the garden a secret from him as Tina became most animated recalling the care and expertise the paramedics had shown.

This incident seemed to sound an alert throughout the neighborhood as friends I had not seen in many months began to show their concern by bringing over a loaf of fresh baked bread or a casserole for my family. Renewed interest in my health was most encouraging. Jeff was pleased that neighbors were concerned and would be checking on us while he was away at work. He was also in discussions with the company to arrange more time at home in order to give me more personal care.

Pastor Murphy and his wife came by occasionally, especially when Jeff was out of town. His wife got down on the children's level and played board games with them so Jeremy and Tina felt she was a great lady, and she was. She made sure that our children were included in activities of the Junior Department. The kids were pretty excited when she got a group of six other kids their ages and took them out to the ice cream shop for an evening of fun. I learned enduring friendships were hard to find for myself and my children and we must nurture them while we could.

The next chemo treatment wiped me out completely. I became so weak it was an effort to lift a spoon and my crippled hands weren't cooperating. It was impossible to eat without spilling some food on my clothes. I tried liquid foods such as broth that can be indulged with a straw, but soon tired of it.

When I was hungry and alone it would often take so much time and effort to get situated where I could reach the food it wasn't worth it. Most of the time it had been hot when left on my nightstand but quite cold by the time I felt like eating. I lacked strength to shuffle to the kitchen and reheat the food in the microwave so it would sit on the nightstand until some kind soul took it away.

Now I understood what Jackie went through - why so much food, thoughtfully prepared and brought to her, was left untouched. Most food had lost its flavor and she had lost her appetite, and then there was the constant vomiting to contend with.

People began badgering me about eating – the children, Jeff and even neighbors. "You have to eat," they would tell me. I tried Jello.™ I tried broth. I tried coleslaw and potato soup, both favorites. I tried ice cream and sherbet. Even rice pudding, another favorite, had lost its flavor. Almost all foods had become bland. I discovered that Popsicles™ were flavorful however they were not a great source of nutrition.

Why would I want to eat tasteless food, especially since it brought with it wretched vomiting? Regardless of what well-meaning people thought, I did try to eat but vomiting became a tiresome pastime. It robbed me of any strength I may have had and left me with a hollow feeling in my stomach. I overheard someone say, "She shouldn't give up so easily." Was I giving up? At the time I didn't think so, but perhaps I was.

During the long days I drifted in and out of sleep as I lay in bed where I was confined the greater part of any day. A few months ago it had been easy to sleep through the night, but not now. I felt if I closed my eyes in sleep, I might not awaken again and I didn't want to go yet - not now. There was still a thread of hope cancer would go into remission and I could get on with my life. I had become consumed with the thought of returning to a state of wellness and normal living.

> "I will both lay me down in peace, and sleep; for thou, Lord only maketh me dwell in safety."
> Psalm 4:8

When one is not well, it's often difficult to give-in to sleep. My trouble was that I had difficulty shutting my mind down. As the cancer advanced, I would lie in a comfortable bed, struggling to keep my eyes open until they would finally droop with fatigue. Somehow I felt if I closed my eyes I might not see another sunrise and I wanted so much to rise from the bed of affliction and be a good wife and mother again.

I knew about a child who had his first asthma attack during the night. His stomach was heaving in and out rapidly as he gasped intermittently for breath. Never having witnessed an asthma attack, his mother had no idea what was happening to her little 5-year-old. She tried to cuddle him, but he kept slipping off her lap onto the floor where he sat on his knees and arched his back for relief. She whispered over and over to him, "Why don't you try to get some sleep?" He whispered, "No mommy, I might not wake up."

She realized her little boy was too frightened to sleep. And now I was feeling like that little boy - staring at the bedroom ceiling, afraid to close my eyes.

Reader, why should you be tormented by fear, which robs you of needed sleep, when the Lord has promised to keep you safely through the night? You may be tormented by fear which is not of God; it is from our adversary, the devil, who only wants to destroy you.

You are God's child and He cares for you more wonderfully than any parent could care for his/her children. When night falls, say a little prayer to commit your life into the keeping of the Lord. Sleep with the peace of God in your heart, knowing Jesus is watching over you with tender care.

As I lay wakeful upon the bed I could hear Jeff breathing soundly across the room. A few months ago I suggested he might be more comfortable sleeping on the couch in the sitting area at the end of our room. This change would enable him to get needed rest without being disturbed by my restlessness.

Why can't I get well so I can be a good wife to him? I wondered what his most innermost thoughts might be as day by day, he watched me getting skinnier and weaker. The pretty wife he married in his youth had changed so much! Cancer had taken its toll on me. I was no fool. When I saw my image in the mirror, a haggard and weary lady looked back at me.

As the night lingered on I might still be wide awake and my thoughts turned to the children. What do they think when they see me wasting away? Do they know I may someday go away and leave them? Surely it has become a heavy burden for them as they are forced to fend for themselves much of the time.

Sleepless nights were not good for me as I dwelt on things over which I had no control. After awhile I would be overcome with sorrow and grief. It felt like I was stranded on an island with the vast ocean stretching out before me and I wasn't able to find the bridge that would take me to the mainland. Erratic thoughts raced through my mind in the dead of night. If I continued to entertain these thoughts, I might soon be weeping. I needed desperately to get back on the rock where I would be safe in Jesus.

I needed to live one day at a time and be strong for whatever waited for me around the corner. I had to be peaceful and joyous for my family in the last few days or weeks I may have on this earth. I determined to get completely off the teeter-totter and have some sense of balance in my life.

To encourage myself I often began to mentally recite scriptures I had known from childhood. The Word of God has power to comfort and inspiration to lift one up.

Some of the scriptures that ministered to me in my desperate time of need were:

"Ask and it shall be given to you; seek and you shall find; knock and it shall be opened unto you".
Matt. 7:7
"God is our refuge and strength, a very present help in time of trouble." Psalms 46:1
"Let not your heart be troubled: ye believe in God, believe also in Me." John 14:1

Before cancer became a reality, breakfast had been a special time with Jeremy and Tina. As mentioned before, I love being a mother. On school mornings, the children would bounce into the kitchen, bantering back and forth cheerily about something or other. I tried to serve something different every morning: it might be French toast, pancakes, eggs and toast or oatmeal. And there was always a glass of orange juice before they boarded the bus for school. Now there were times I saw sadness in their eyes and felt they needed more time for recreation, away from the house and sickness.

Long days alone in the house become boring. I wished for friendship. My circle of friends used to call frequently and we would enjoy intelligent conversation, keeping up-to-date on local happenings. Further, I missed fun lunches with them after which we would go shopping together at the mall in the city.

As the disease progressed my friends seemed to retreat more and more. I'm still wondering if they thought cancer was contagious. While I'm sure they hadn't forgotten me, I wondered if perhaps they just didn't know what they could possibly say to make me feel better.

I felt desperate for someone to call on the phone again or to receive a note from someone in my church family. It would only take a few moments for a friend to send a humorous card to put a smile on my face. And if someone would knock on my door for a surprise visit it would simply be delightful.

Joy happens when we take the time to care about someone other than ourselves. Joy returns to us when someone we've blessed thanks us with misty eyes.

My thoughts turned to my cousin Eddie and I wondered how he was coping in his bout with cancer. Was he surrounded with friends for moral support? Jeff called Eddie after dinner. He had just finished a radiation treatment and seemed to be in fairly good spirits. He asked to talk with me. He was curious to know if I had lost my hair, so I mentioned the lovely wig I was wearing.

Though I had never seen Eddie with more than a wisp of hair on top of his head, he said he was now as bald as a bowling ball and he wasn't planning on shopping for a hairpiece. I was delighted to learn he had not yet experienced any bouts of vomiting.

Eddie was also experiencing sleepless nights, often lying in bed wondering if he would ever be normal again. Though his doctor was optimistic about his recovery, he wondered how much time he might have. Like me, he'd think about the possibility and wonder how it would happen. Would he simply go to sleep and not awaken again? Or would he be in a hospital bed with oxygen and drips and so forth? We talked about passing from this life to our eternal rewards - surely it would be a most joyous experience!

I knew Jesus would guide me through Heaven's gates and Eddie felt the same, so it really didn't matter, but there was a nagging fear of the unknown for both of us. We were chatting as though we expected to lose the battle we were waging against cancer. Eddie said a brief prayer for me and we said goodnight. Jeff and I chatted awhile about Eddie's battle with cancer. Then he reminded me of a scripture in Ecclesiastes 3:1,2:

> *"To everything there is a season, a time for every purpose under heaven: a time to be born and a time to die."*

Before closing my eyes in sleep I prayed for Eddie's return to good health.

> *Peace lies within your family. Make the most of every moment you have with them. Your loved ones need to see you at peace. They understand the mental and emotional battle you are waging for a return to health. Learn to smile, even when you don't feel like it.*

There is always hope that you may turn the corner and go into remission, and many of you will. What a glad day that will be! Take comfort in knowing many friends and relatives are praying for you.

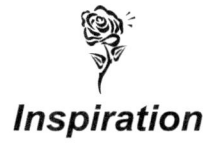

Inspiration

"The angel of the Lord encampeth 'round about them that fear Him and delivereth them."
Psalm 34:7

Application

In the New Testament we read about an angel who was dispatched to 'trouble the water' in the Pool of Bethesda. Persons who were impotent, blind, lame, etc. lay beside the pool waiting for the angel to come and trouble the waters. Those who stepped into the water would be healed – made perfectly whole.

Angels were sent to Jesus when he knelt in the garden of Gethsemane. He was agonizing in prayer, knowing He was about to be delivered up to be crucified. Father God saw the agony His son was in and sent an angel to strengthen Jesus for the suffering He would soon endure.

If our spiritual eyes could be opened, very possibly we might see angels protecting us from harm and danger night and day. How wonderful to know God loves us so much He dispatches angels to watch over us continually.

O LORD, YOU ARE MY GOD.
I WILL EXTOL YOU.

I WILL PRAISE YOUR NAME

FOR YOU HAVE DONE WONDERFUL THINGS.

YOUR COUNSELS OF OLD ARE FAITHFULNESS

AND TRUTH.

YOU HAVE BEEN A STRENGTH

TO THE POOR,

A REFUGE FROM THE STORM,

AND A SHADE FROM THE HEAT.....

FROM ISAIAH 25

6

Pretending

It was our wedding anniversary and Jeff had left a note on my bathroom mirror. "Happy Anniversary! Golden Swan. Tonight. 7 o'clock. Home early." Sweet Jeff, it was like him to remember our anniversary. We always celebrated in a special way. The Golden Swan was our favorite restaurant overlooking the Pacific. One could sit at a table with a commanding view of the tide rolling onto the beach. To top it off, a wandering violinist might entertain us with a wonderful classical piece.

It was really exciting to know we would be going out, but I wasn't sure I could pull it off. It would take more strength than I had to get dressed for an evening out. However, I knew in my heart this could be our last anniversary so it was important to make every effort to have a great time for Jeff's sake.

With Tina's help I was seated in front of the open closet in my room in order to select a dress suitable for the occasion. The 54 pounds I had lost were not kind to me. "What am I going to do," I wondered under my breath. Sensing my frustration, Tina retrieved several pretty dresses from the closet and held them up for my nod of approval. Finally Tina showed me a lovely shrimp pink chiffon dress. It might be one that could be 'doctored' to fit my slender body. A favorite, it had silver rhinestones inset on the bodice. A matching chiffon jacket would complement the dress. I told Tina this would be the one, while secretly I wondered if perhaps I would be overdressed for our little town. If we were going out in the city, the dress would be perfect. Oh well, I thought, I can wear what I want – after all, it's my anniversary!

Tina was so sweet. I thought perhaps this was the perfect time to have a little chat, one I had been dreading.

She and her brother too, needed to be prepared in the event I should not survive this ordeal.

"Tina, you're a very perceptive young lady and surely you've noticed that I'm not getting better. Chemo isn't working for me as hoped." Tina reached out to touch me, "Mom you don't have to...." and her voice trailed off. "Yes, hon, I need to tell you how proud I am of you. You have taken over many of my responsibilities since I became ill. It doesn't seem fair that you should be burdened with caring for me as well as keeping things running somewhat normally around the house. Life isn't always fair. I know now that I may not be a survivor." Tina chimed in, "Mom please don't talk like that. You can get better, I know you can."

"I know it's not easy to discuss the possibility of my passing, but we need to think about it," I announced lamely as my chin quivered with emotion. "You have studies to do, so go on now, and we'll continue this discussion later." Tina reached down and we embraced for a few moments before she left the room.

I sat on the edge of the bed contemplating our anniversary and a night out – it had been a long time since Jeff and I had gone to dinner. I was feeling somewhat apprehensive, but I knew in my heart I must make this occasion special for him.

Jeff arrived home from work and came to assist me. It was a special treat to sit in the shower again. Jeff dried me off and walked me to the dressing table. I looked for makeup that might fill in some of the wrinkles in my once-pretty face. I applied a little peach color to my cheeks and selected a delicate peach shade of lipstick. Could I detect a little improvement in my appearance? Maybe I should do this every day.

The lovely chiffon was draped over me and I stood to get a full view in the mirror. Jeff stepped forward to adjust my wig. I wasn't prepared for the sight of the lady who looked back at me. She easily looked twice my age. Reduced to skin and bones, it would take two of me to fill out the dress. Unable to suppress my emotions, I fell across the bed and cried my heart out. Jeff wanted to know what the problem was and he began to offer realistic solutions.

"Why not wear a belt to take up the slack," he suggested as he reached into a drawer and began to hand me belts of all descriptions. Nothing was right, that is, until he found a rhinestone belt. Jeff gently put the belt around my waist, smoothing the extra fullness into neat little folds, like pleats, under the belt. When he finished, the effect was okay - not terrific, but okay.

My sweet Jeff helped me get seated at the vanity again. He told me to close my eyes, a hint that something special was about to happen. I obeyed him and waited expectantly. Soon something cool touched my neck and I knew Jeff had bought me some jewelry. He bent over and kissed me as my eyes opened to discover a beautiful silver chain with an attached gorgeous sapphire pendant. "Oh, Jeff, it's simply beautiful! I love the deep blue shade of the stone. It complements my dress perfectly! You make me feel very special!" "You are special, my dear," he replied as he reached out to hug me tight. Looking about my dressing table, I spotted my favorite perfume. After a puff of fragrance, we were now ready for a night out.

Jeff took my arm and we went to say goodnight to Jeremy and Tina who sweetly complimented me on my appearance. They may have sensed my reticence to go out. They seemed excited to see me dressed up. Tina took a moment to brush a finger across the pendant before she insisted, "Scat; get outta here and have some fun."

Seated in the restaurant, Jeff reached across the table and caressed my hand. He could see I needed a little support and moved his chair next to mine. Now I could rest my head on his shoulder occasionally. It was such a gracious gesture as it had become difficult to hold my head up. The vast ocean stretched out before us. Waves gently swept ashore. The wet, sandy beach glistened in the moonlight. Oh, how I wished this moment would never end!

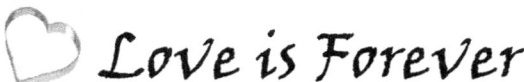 Love is Forever

Jeff, it's so wonderful to be out of the house. You can't know how good it is to be here with you - just the two of us on our anniversary." Jeff squeezed my hand, but he said he didn't feel much like talking. He just looked at me. "Honey, have I told you lately how much I love you," I asked my husband and very best friend in the world. "And I you," was his quick reply. He squeezed my tiny, delicate hand again and continued, "From the moment I met you my life has been complete and full of much happiness – more than I could ever express in words."

The waiter was standing at our table, but I hardly knew what to order. Food could wait; I just wanted to enjoy the happiness of these few moments with Jeff, aware it may be our last wedding anniversary.

Jeff sensed my hesitation and suggested trout for my entrée. The mild fish would not be too filling. I wasn't used to eating real meals anymore and mostly just moved the food around on my plate while Jeff finished his prime rib and lobster. The effort of the evening was exhausting me but I couldn't spoil our special evening out for my sweet Jeff.

My gift to Jeff was something he had admired more than once in a jewelry store window. Now it was my turn to do something special for him. I reached into my handbag for a little box which had been beautifully wrapped for the occasion. "Jeff, I have something for you," I murmured softly as I placed the gift before him. He looked at me with a question, "How did you…." "I asked Tex to pick it up for me." Jeff was quick to remove the wrapping and open the box. The expression on his face when he saw the wide gold band with the gorgeous tiger eye stone was worth the effort of going out.

A Promise Kept

When Jeff and I repeated our wedding vows 15 years ago, we promised to love and care for each other 'for richer or for poorer; in sickness and in health.'

Neither of us could have dreamed then that cancer would strain our relationship. In wonderful ways, my loyal Jeff had demonstrated his enduring love and care for me. Our sincere marriage vows had carried us through this exhausting trial.

Jeff was always there when I needed him. Sometimes he anticipated what I needed before I had it figured out. Though he had never been around someone with terminal disease, he had a special sensitivity that I appreciated. Jeff was precious!

Anniversaries are always special, but this one was extra special for us. And it wasn't over yet, for Jeff promised I would have another surprise the following day. I began to guess what it might be, but he would laugh and say I was way off-base.

Dinner was over and we moved to the deck for awhile. The violinist meandered to the deck as he played strains of a special love song. We sat quietly on a bench holding hands, watching the waves gently come ashore. Leaning my head on Jeff's broad shoulder I relaxed to the rhythmic and hypnotic movement of the moonlit water. We didn't need to talk. It was enough to be together for this special time of remembrance. I felt I could stay here forever. Silvery moonlight danced like diamonds upon the crest of each wave as it spread out on the beach. When we stood to leave I turned too quickly, lost my balance and began to fall, but Jeff was quick to catch me. What would I ever do without him?

Driving home Jeff told me again of the happiness and contentment he had felt in our marriage and how much it hurt to see me suffer day after day.

The following afternoon I heard Jeremy and Tina come in from school and begin arguing about something in the front part of the house. Managing to get out of bed, I slipped into my scuffs, grabbed my cane and began gliding across the room for my robe. I had to know what the ruckus was all about and try to calm the children down.

Before I could get my robe I saw Jeremy coming toward me pushing a wheelchair. "What is going on," I gasped "and where did you get the wheelchair?"

"Mom, this is another anniversary surprise Dad got for you, but he made us promise not to tell. It has just been delivered and we have been arguing over who is going to push you around the house. Isn't this the greatest? Well, don't look so surprised, Mom. With this chair you can gain some of your independence again – you can get out of your room and spend more time with us." Jeremy was persuasive but I wasn't sure I wanted to be pushed around.

Tina bounced out of the chair and stood in front of me. "May I help you into your carriage ma'am," she asked brightly, curtsying in her cute little way. Both of my children were showing their affection and care. "Well, this is totally unexpected! I never dreamed of getting around in my own wheelchair!

"Now I can go out onto the patio. Tell me, is it necessary for me to be pushed or can I operate it by myself," I asked. Jeremy excitedly began to explain how to use my new wheels. I could not disappoint my family. I could see what a great gift this chair would be. With these wheels I could have a better quality of life when alone in the house. I could put away the cane and walker.

Jeff and the children had put a lot of attention on me and been most patient and sweet in spite of the ordeal we had all been experiencing. Feeling special and spoiled, I made another resolve to get well.

The 84 pounds I was carrying around wasn't enough to put flesh on my bones. I wanted so much to gain weight, but if I couldn't digest food and keep it down, I would continue to lose weight and get weaker and weaker. At times the doctor refused to give me a chemo treatment until I could gain a few pounds. I appreciated his consideration, but I knew it may not make any difference in the outcome.

It wasn't fun to look into the mirror anymore. The pretty face I used to see looking back at me was no longer there. Weight loss had created deep wrinkles in my face and my darkened eyes seem to have gravitated to my navel.

My current physical state must have been tremendously difficult for both Jeff and the children. There were times I was so weak it was impossible to get out of bed in a normal fashion. I had to carefully roll to the carpeted floor and crawl to the bathroom. What an ordeal that was! Even then I usually couldn't make it to the bathroom in time and ended up with vomit on my nightgown or pajamas and, of course, the carpet.

The doctor never told me to expect situations such as this. How could I get out of this predicament, I wondered? This was terribly discouraging if I let myself think about it.

However there were some better days along the way. As the days became longer I made every effort to fill the time with good memories. Tina had brought scrapbooks from previous vacations and special celebrations to my room. If I felt like sitting in a chair at a small table near the bed, I could take my time remembering fun we had together as a family. Entertaining myself in this manner lifted my spirits. Pleasant memories are good for the soul.

If I was having a bad day (soon after chemo) I couldn't welcome visitors to my room. I probably didn't have my wig on and didn't want anyone to see me. As I said earlier, I responded to a knock on the bedroom door with "Don't come in; no you can't come in!" Memories may linger with the children and friends a long time and they should be good memories.

In spite of my new "wheels," I rarely got out of the bedroom due to the negative effects chemo continued to thrust upon my body. One might think the chemo must be working, bringing me back to health, but such was not the case. Chemo was not doing its job as intended. Lately Dr. Unruh hadn't had any encouraging lab report and he was somewhat mute when I asked when chemo might 'kick in.' I kept hoping for exciting news, however I read the expression in his eyes and knew he did not have much hope for my return to health. .

Jeremy and Tina knew there needed to be changes at home. They had a meeting with their father and told him we needed a nurse for mom and secondly, a house-keeper who could also cook. Jeff assured them he had already been looking into the situation and we would have some help in a day or so.

Unknown to me or the children, Jeff had engaged the services of an agency that would recruit and check out references of potential housekeepers. We needed someone with 3-way experience as they would become cook, housekeeper and nurse.

Two days later Jeff came to my bedside and held out a box containing a lovely satin robe and matching satin scuffs. He knew how much I liked pink and they were just perfect. He helped me shower and dress in the pink robe before whisking me up in his arms and depositing me, like a bag of potatoes, into the soft chaise lounge which had become a favorite place for me. What would I do without my man? He is most perceptive, always thinking ahead to what I may need.

"What's going on," I inquired before Jeff told me he had a very special surprise for me. Jeremy and Tina were giggling and looking at each other. They kept looking into the kitchen as though they were expecting someone.

"Jeff, I don't understand what's going on. Where's the surprise?" "It's in the kitchen hon. I'll go get it now," he replied as he headed for the kitchen. I don't know exactly what I expected to see, but in a few moments the kitchen's dutch door opened and a wonderful warm – big and grand German lady burst upon my vision. "Hon, this is Erika, our new housekeeper." She was an angel sent from God

Erika was dressed in a navy blue uniform adorned with a crisp white collar and cuffs at the sleeves. Her apron was crisp and white. She wore dark cotton hosiery and practical shoes – good for being on one's feet. Her gray hair was pulled back into a wide bun. She had a smile as big as the crescent moon spread across her face.

I fell in love with her immediately. She told me of her past experience as a practical nurse. Further, she enjoyed housework and cooking, especially 'good German food.' With misty eyes I welcomed Erika into our home.

Excerpts from Revelation 22:

- And he showed me a pure river of water of life, clear as crystal, proceeding from the throne of God and of the Lamb.

- In the middle of the street, and on either side of the river, was the tree of life, which bore twelve fruits, each tree yielding its fruit every month. And the leaves of the tree were for the healing of the nations..

- And there shall be no more curse, but the throne of God and of the Lamb shall be in it and His servants shall serve Him.

- And there shall be no night there: They need no lamp nor light of the sun, for the Lord God gives them light. And they shall reign forever and ever.

- Blessed are those that do His commandments that they may have the right to the tree of life, and may enter through the gates into the city.

7

Saying Goodbye

Eighteen months had passed since the day I initially heard the three life-threatening words, "*You have cancer.*" Jeremy had the flu and was forced to stay home from school for three days. My motherly instinct got me into my marvelous wheels in order to check on him. I hadn't used my new mode of transportation often, but it surely was a blessing when I needed it.

Erika was at his bedside taking his temperature. When she finished I asked her to make a cup of hot tea with honey to relieve his sore throat. Jeremy was bleary eyed with a red nose. "Mom, you shouldn't be up waiting on me. I'll be okay," he asserted as I sat on the edge of his bed wiping his brow.

I forgot about my fragile immune system as I wanted so much to play mother again. He needed care and I could easily give him medicine to curb the cough. I certainly wasn't a very frisky nurse bustling about, but he did get some attention.

In a few days I developed a cold, which soon advanced to a gut-wrenching cough and finally the doctor admitted me to the hospital with pneumonia.

The ambulance arrived with sirens blaring to announce an emergency. Jeff chose to ride in the ambulance with me. He held my tiny wrinkled hand and rubbed it between his strong athletic hands. He didn't speak; his eyes were misty and he was deep in serious thought. As I lay there, my mind was racing. "Am I going to die? I don't want to die. Not now." My eyes were also misty as the ambulance arrived at the hospital.

Two nurses were assigned to my care. They hovered over me like a mother hen, setting up oxygen to assist me in breathing. They proceeded to poke my arms and install several intravenous drips. Oh, how I hated those things! Once my vital signs had been taken and recorded, Jeff came close to my bedside. He took my hand and assured me he would be staying with me. If I needed anything, I should let him know and he would ring for a nurse.

Jeff knew the Bible well and he was always ready to share the Word when needed. It certainly was needed now. With his hand on my forehead he began to recite a familiar portion from the 91st chapter of Psalms.

> *"He that dwelleth in the secret place of the Most High shall abide under the shadow of the Almighty. I will say of the Lord, He is my refuge and my fortress: my God, in Him will I trust. Surely He shall deliver thee from the snare of the fowler, and from the noisome pestilence. He shall cover thee with His feathers and under His wings shalt thou trust."*

Looking up into Jeff's face, I noticed he was misty-eyed again. My steady, sweet Jeff had choked up a little as he was reading. He had been a real tower of strength for me and the children during this trial of all trials. He was the most wonderful man I had ever known. God could not have given me a more perfect husband and I hoped he felt the same about me. I knew I would never return home to my family. I wanted him to remember the happy times we had shared and our love that had endured the rugged ordeal of coping with terminal illness.

I was tired and closed my eyes to sleep. When I awoke, it was morning. Jeff wasn't there. The nurse told me he had stayed by my side until 5 o'clock in the morning when he went home for a little sleep.

One of my brothers was sitting in a corner chair. He must have come in while I was sleeping. He walked to the foot of the bed, greeted me with his traditional greeting, "Hi Sis," and began to tickle my toes. As a result of chemo, there was no longer any feeling in them. He looked somewhat disappointed that I had not reacted to his effort to bring a smile to my face. It had been months since I had seen him and it would have been a treat to be able to sit up and visit.

It was good to see him, but it made me somewhat uneasy. Obviously, someone had called him. Did that mean the medical staff anticipated I may pass on soon?

My brother sensed I didn't have much strength for visiting, so after a few minutes he politely excused himself and went to the hospital cafeteria.

At noon, a nurse was sitting beside my bed trying to feed me when my brother showed up again. He made an effort to get my mind off my dismal situation by saying funny things to get me to laugh. I was too weak to respond, however, and just looked at him with a blank stare. As I began to gag on the thin applesauce, he suggested to the nurse that perhaps he could take over the job of feeding me. However, he wasn't any more successful at getting me to eat because I was afraid food might induce vomiting again. He took the tray of food from the room and I didn't see him for about an hour.

Jeff arranged with his company to spend most of his time with me. Of course, he brought Jeremy and Tina with him which pleased me greatly. The children looked sad and hardly knew what to say. I felt they, too, did not expect me to return home. Though I knew my family was with me until visiting hours were over, it was impossible to stay awake. It was an effort to breathe and I just simply needed to rest. I wanted so much to be able to visit with them, but I'm sure they understood when my eyelids kept closing.

When I awoke the following morning, nurses were taking my vital signs and whispering quietly among themselves. Jeff had fallen asleep in a chair. The activity wakened him and he excused himself, promising to return after breakfast. The nurses dressed me in a fresh gown and changed the bedding. One of them situated my wig and helped me apply a little eyebrow pencil and lipstick. I knew I must look dreadful and was thankful the nurses would pretty me up a bit.

I appreciated the dedication of the entire hospital staff that cared for me. Their attention to detail was proof of their calling to the field of medicine.

It was almost 10 AM when I felt a touch on my shoulder and opened my eyes to see my good friend, Tex. "Oh, Tex, it's so good to see you," I gasped breathlessly. She looked the absolute picture of health. She must have come from the beauty salon as her lovely red hair was perfectly styled.

I had not seen Tex for several weeks. She reached for my hand and I told her how happy I was for her healing. She knew how desperately I longed to recover and she prayed for me.

Jeff came in while Tex was praying. When she finished, she broke into tears and quickly left the room. Jeff followed her into the hall where they chatted for a few moments. Then he returned to my side and we were alone. I wanted to know about Jeremy and Tina. How were they coping? Had they adjusted to having Erika in the house? He was quick to acknowledge everything was running smoothly at home. I was glad. My family had struggled to maintain some sense of order for a long time.

Jeff received a call on his cell phone. In order not to disturb me, he went into the hallway for a short discussion with someone from his office. My heart was heavy and I felt sad for him. Knowing that the cancer had been advancing all along, and now with complications of pneumonia, I felt it might be just a matter of minutes before I would part from him. Jeff may have felt the same as he stayed with me until late in the night.

My thoughts overwhelmed me and I felt like crying but my eyes were dry. Pastor Murphy walked into the room. He observed my anxiety and reached out to comfort me. Before he could say anything, I blurted out, "Why...is...this...hap...pen...ing...to...me? What...have ...I...done? Will I...ever...go...home... again?" Before he...could...re...spond...to...my...plea,..I...con...tinued, "I love...Jeff...and...the...children...so...much...I don't ...want...to...leave...them...not...now...Life...is... precious ...Why...have...I been...tormented...by...cancer? I have...tried... to...live ... pleas...ing to...the... Lord."

Pastor pulled a chair close to my bed and leaned toward me. In a gentle voice he assured me that I had nothing to do with the onset of the disease. He explained how many things happen to us in this life and we have no explanation for the 'why.' Through all our trials, the Lord has promised to be with us. Pastor Murphy leaned closer and whispered that he felt the Lord may be calling me to my eternal home. He said I would be in Jesus' presence with loved ones who were waiting for me. There was nothing to fear for the Lord Jesus would send his angels to carry me to Heaven. I would take one last step from the dusty roads of Earth and step onto streets of gold in my eternal home. He told me I would be beautiful, perfect and whole in the Lord's presence. Then he prayed a comforting prayer for me before he left to visit other patients.

A few minutes later one of my sisters from a bordering state, along with a very special lady and her husband, came to my bedside. I was somewhat startled to see them. Then I knew my family had been notified to come quickly if they wanted to see me before I would pass from this life. Smiling broadly, my sister leaned down to plant a kiss gently on my cheek as she greeted me with "Hi there." I was thrilled to see her.

I wanted to rise from the bed and serve her a delicious tea in a China cup. The lady who brought my sister prepared a dish of thin warm cereal she knew I could probably digest. She was always so good to me! She had to leave soon to pick up her children at school, but promised to return later.

Finally the room was quiet. My sister squeezed my arm and began chatting about her flight. It was a one-way conversation as she could see how tired I was. At this point, I only had strength to speak a few words at a time. She placed a chair by the window and began to softly sing an old hymn of the faith I knew so well. "*I need thee, oh I need thee. Every hour I need thee. Oh bless me now my Savior; I come to thee.*" *(Annie S. Hawkes, author)*

It was like a breath of fresh air, just what I needed. I had always enjoyed hearing my sister sing. She had been soloist for all our family weddings and special occasions and gospel conventions, etc. She sensed I needed my rest. With my eyes closed tightly, I enjoyed the sweet, soft music. After awhile I heard harmony and opened my eyes to discover a brother-in-law sitting at the foot of the bed. Their voices blended well. His wife (another sister) had a bad head cold and was smart to stay home.

During the next few hours other family members came. Some of them had driven many hours and must have been exhausted. Obviously it was time for final good-byes. My family is deeply religious so there was lots of scripture reading and soft harmonious singing of favorite gospel songs in the room. It was good to see them, but I was so weak I could only lean back on the pillow and rest with my eyes closed, just drifting in and out.

Other visitors came during evening visiting hours. Jeff brought Jeremy, Tina and Erika too. My beautiful family stood at my bedside, but it was evident they didn't know what to say. I felt their love and concern as they touched me gently or kissed me on the cheek, and words didn't seem necessary at a time such as this. After a few moments, they could sense I was struggling just to breathe and some of them said goodbye and left the room. I knew they would be huddled together in the family waiting room down the hall.

The closeness of family and friends at a time such as this is so precious! I was sorry I couldn't get up and be the gracious hostess I would like to be. As I was thinking these thoughts, I drifted off to sleep and had a most wonderful dream. I cannot explain it, but this dream dramatically changed my attitude about an end-of-life experience.

Prior to this, I admit I mostly felt sorry for myself and often questioned why God would let this happen to me. Why would a loving God take me from my family who needed me? I didn't want to die. I was fighting to live. There was so much to live for. I didn't want to leave Jeff and Jeremy and Tina. I had been clinging to life with all that was in me, but now I knew what the REAL FUTURE held for me! This wonderful and exciting dream had radically changed my views on dying.

Reader, if the Lord takes you home, it doesn't mean He hasn't heard the faithful prayers of family and friends who yearn to see you recover from illness and disease. Family and friends need to know the Lord has a specific plan for each of us. That plan may include your home-going. In the present we may not see clearly, but our Lord does all things well – and we don't question Him.

I awoke from the dream to discover I was back in the hospital room. Nurses hovered about, checking my pulse and blood pressure. They looked concerned. As I opened my eyes, their faces brightened, "Well hello, we thought we lost you." However, I was disappointed. The dream had been so realistic, I thought the Lord had permanently transported me to my new heavenly home.

My finite imagination could never have envisioned the beauty of Heaven in any proportion of reality. Many times I had read descriptive text in the book of Revelation (last book in the Bible) about heaven, and wondered about how it would feel to be in the presence of God. Now the Lord had opened my consciousness to the reality of seeing Him, of worshipping Him, of the vast beauty and peace beyond compare. Heaven suddenly seemed very real and I sincerely wanted to go there.

The grandeur of heaven is indescribable. I'm a woman who loves precious gems and I saw them all around the City of God. Can you believe streets of pure gold and crystal streams? There were many gates; each one was one radiant pearl. A few of the gems I saw were jasper, sapphire, emerald, and topaz Having had a little peek into my final home through this dream, it was especially disappointing to discover I was back in the hospital.

I was now ready to go be with the Lord forever. Fellowship with my Lord was what I longed for more than anything. I longed to be free of my wretched body and be beautiful and whole again! "Oh, Jesus, I'm ready to go!" The awesome feeling I had experienced in my dream had transformed me. The dream was so real and I wanted to share it. I no longer had a fear of passing from life on earth to my eternal home in Heaven. In fact, I had a new expectancy of going Home to be with my Lord and Savior Jesus Christ!

The nurse supervisor found Jeff in the family waiting room and called him to come quickly if he wanted to say a last goodbye. He rushed into the room with family members, looking genuinely concerned. My wonderful husband pulled a chair close to the bed and kissed me on the cheek. It was so good to have him by my side at this momentous time. Pneumonia had weakened me so that it was difficult to talk, but I had to share my new and exhilarating experience with Jeff. I motioned for him to lean closer. With some effort I was able to recount my visit to heaven.

"Jeff," I whispered, "I have...had...a...vision... or... a...dream...I'm...not...sure...but... I've...been... with... Jesus. I...can't...begin...to...tell...you...how...wonder ...ful...it...was. I...was...in...this...beau...ti...ful place ...too...spec...tac...u..lar...to...de...scribe... An...angel came...to...take..me...to...Jesus... He...was...seated...

...on...a...glist'ning...gold...en....throne...I was ...in... the...pres...ence...of...God. Je...sus...lift...ed His arms ...toward... me...invit...ing... me... to...come...to...Him. And there...was...worship...and...sing...ing...such...as ...I've...never...heard...be...fore... Jeff... it...was...won ...der...ful...and...glor...ious... Can you... im...agine... crys...tal...foun...tains...and...streets...of...pure gold? Best...of...all... I've... been...with... Je...sus.... He... told...me...if...I'm...faithful...I...shall...soon...be... with ... Him... Honey...the...Lord...has...let me ...know...He ...will...take...me...home ...soon...to...be...with...Him... Now I'm...not afraid...anymore...to die."

Jeff leaned over and kissed my forehead, "Honey that is the most marvelous dream you've had of heaven and it does seem to have given you a new measure of peace, but I can't give you up. We have a whole lifetime ahead of us. Surely you will get better. You must know I can't live without you! Certainly we all want God's will for you, but if He chooses to take you home, it will mean emptiness for me.

"I need you by my side. You are my life. You help me have balance in my life. And I know Jeremy and Tina feel the same way. It's so good to see you excited and radiant after having a vision or dream of heaven. To see the Lord is a marvelous treat one would not soon forget. I can't imagine the feeling you must have had to be in the presence of almighty deity. I'm thankful for the dream you've had as it has lifted your spirits."

Jeff was interrupted as a few more family members left the room one by one. There was probably a lot of talking going on in the hallway due to the frustration of the advancement of the disease. I was glad when they left the room so I might have this time alone with Jeff and the children.
I needed to tell them one last time how much I loved them and was thankful for the love and concern they had given me throughout this abominable ordeal. Each of them felt an urge to respond directly to me. As good as I could, I managed to put some words together, though it was all I could do as I was very short of breath. "It's...wonder...ful...to...hear...you...say...such...kind... things...but ...I...am...tired. Can...cer...has...gotten the... best...of...me...and...I can't...fight...any...more. I...have... no...dig...ni...ty...or... qual...i...ty ...of... life ...left. Un...til...now...I've...been...clinging... to...life

…with a…vengeance… I hav…en't… wanted…to…go away…and leave…you. I must…tell…you about…a… wonder…ful… dream…I had…today. I was…in …heaven…with…Jesus… He…told…me I…would …be …with…Him…soon…if…I…am… faithful…I…will …try …to…de…scribe…my…dream…of…hea…ven…I…saw … Je…sus…He…spoke…to…me.

Hea…ven…is…so…beau…ti…ful…I..wish…you…could …see…it…too…Now…I'm…not…afraid…to…die…for..I …know…Je…sus…will…meet…me…at…the…pearly… gates…of…the…gold…en…city. I'm rea…dy …now …to…go…to…my…heavenly…home… when…Jesus… sends…His…an…gel.….for…me…Don't…cry …or… be …sad…because…I…will…have…a…new…body. There …won't…be…any…can…cer…in…Heav'n… I…won't… feel…any…more…pain."

My dear loved ones stood silently with tears in their eyes. Jeff picked up the conversation by saying "Your mom has had a wonderful vision or dream today. It seems that Jesus has shown her just a little taste of what Heaven will be like."

Coming to Terms

Dear Lord, You're watching over me.

I know You care for me
and have a plan for my life.
   I submit to that plan now.

I'm tired of struggling to figure things out.
I want to trust You, my Savior and Lord.
I don't want to be afraid, but sometimes I am,
   for without a miracle I shall die.

I don't want to go away from those dear to me
but I can't battle any longer.
You have made a place for me:
   my eternal home up yonder.

You showed me heaven in a dream,
I saw a new and true reality:
Angels will come to fly me away
   Where I'll be sheltered with You eternally!

Tina ran to my bedside and put her face against my cheek. "Don't die, mom; you can't die and leave us." She was sobbing and I wanted so much to hold her tight and whisper in her ear, but my hands were not free due to the intravenous drips.

Jeremy was questioning his dad, "Why has this happened to Mom? I thought chemotherapy was supposed to make Mom well! What's happening, Dad? We can't let her die! How can we get along without her?" His soul was wrenched at the thought of losing me.

Three of the most precious people in my life were grieving at my passing. It was almost more than they could bear. Sweet Jeff, though broken-hearted himself, was doing his best to console our two children. I wanted to shout, "Don't cry for me. I shall be complete and whole in my heavenly home. I will wait for you to come." Looking upon my family one last time I thanked God for them.

Jeff put his arm around Jeremy and did his best to comfort him. "Jeremy, I too, am heartbroken, for I had great hope that Mom would be a survivor. As hard as this is to bear, we must not be bitter or angry. It's true, God does have a plan for each of us. Sometimes we don't like the things that take place in our lives. They can be painful. We have all fought with Mom for her deliverance from cancer, but if the Lord chooses to release her from the pain of cancer by taking her, we must be willing to accept that release."

Jeremy stood with his arms folded defiantly, "But Dad, why didn't the chemo work? I thought the doctor said Mom needed it to get well." "Well son, this is what the doctor told me. He also said there hasn't been enough research into ovarian cancer. He told me some months ago that chemotherapy wasn't having the desired effect on the cancer. At that time, we agreed to try a more aggressive treatment, but for whatever reason, it has not been successful.

"I know how you and Tina feel. I, myself, cannot imagine life without your Mom. She has been my life for 15 years. She has been my happiness, my purpose in living and what I work so hard for. The house is going to seem empty without her. We must remember, though, that when we come into this life there is no guarantee we will live forever. Each day infants, toddlers and teens pass from this life. We will not all live to be 70 or 80."

Jeff continued, "Your Mom is inheriting eternal life and a peace indescribable. She fought to live because she could not bear to part from us. It's time now for us to let her go to the Savior she has loved and served. We must pray for strength to endure the pain of her passing. It won't be easy, but God will help us."

My two darling children were softly weeping. Jeff encircled them in his arms. All three of them were shattered at the rapid pace of events. They weren't prepared for my release from this life. What could I say to ease their pain? Jeff composed himself somewhat and I heard him say, "Your mother is so happy about the thought of entering into Glory that I feel we must share her happiness. This is what we, as Christians, live for: to be in the presence of the Lord. Mom now has a peace I have never known her to have. Look at her radiant face. She is totally transformed. I shall remember her like this, glowing and radiant. Can you do the same?"

Jeff continued, "Mom has fought cancer with all her might. Perhaps this is the way God is answering her prayers, by taking her home. She will never again feel the sensation of pain. Cancer will be eradicated from her body. She will have a **new** body – a **glorified** body in the City of God with her Savior. She will live forever in Jesus' presence. What more could we want for her?"

I motioned for Jeremy to come closer. "Jeremy, I'm...go...ing...to a...won...der...ful...place. I... fought ...dying....for...a....long...time...because...I...did...not... want...to...go...away...and...leave...you. Today...I..had ...the...most...won...der...ful...dream...and...all...the... fear...I...had...is...gone. I know...Je...sus...will... send ...his...an...gel...for...me...and...in... an..in...stant... I'll ...be...in...His... pres...ence. I'll...wait...for...you ... your...sis...ter...and...your...dad..to...come...be ...with ....me. One day...when...it's...God's... time... we... shall...be...to...gether...again. Be...faith ...ful...to... the...Lord...Jeremy. Take...care...of...Tina. .and...stay ...close...to...your...dad... I know...you... will...grow... up ...to...be...a...fine...man...like...your.. father."

Tina moved close and began to stroke my arm. Her eyes were filled with tears as she bent over to kiss me. I wondered how she would manage without me, but I knew in my heart things would work out for her. Tina had many talents for a young girl. She was creative. She was courageous. She was a leader, not a follower.

As the moments went by it became more and more obvious to me my spirit would soon fly to my Heavenly Father. Jeff sensed it as he motioned Jeremy and Tina into the corner of the room where they could sit down. Jeff comforted the children in the best way he knew how. He was overcome with the knowledge that his sweet wife was going to Glory.

With mixed feelings, he reached for the Bible on the nearby cabinet and began to read an appropriate portion of scripture from Revelation, chapter 21:

"And I saw a new heaven and a new earth and I, John saw the holy city, Jerusalem, coming down from God out of heaven, prepared as a bride adorned for her husband. And I heard a great voice out of heaven saying, 'Behold the tabernacle of God is with men, and He will dwell with them and they shall be His people and God Himself shall be with them and be their God. And God shall wipe all tears away from their eyes...' "

These were the last words I heard Jeff say. Suddenly I was again in this wonderful place of my dream, with Jesus forever and ever! It seemed that I could look back into the hospital room and see my body in the bed and my family around me. Nurses began rushing into the room. They took my vital signs again. My family was huddled together at the foot of the bed. Jeff had his arms around my two special children who were weeping.

I wanted to shout at them, "Don't cry for me. If you could see where I am at this very moment, you would be rejoicing with me. Heaven is pure JOY. It is PEACE. There is no feeling like this in all the earth. This is LIFE, **real** LIFE. **Everlasting** LIFE! My body has been ravished by disease, but God has made me whole in an instant. I am standing in the presence of Jesus, who took my place on the cross. I am beautiful again and I feel no pain or anxiety. I'm so thankful I received Him as my Savior so that I can be with Him in heaven for all eternity. I shall wait for you to come when it is your time."

At that moment my spiritual eyes were opened and I understood the full meaning of a verse I'd heard all my adult life and wondered about:

> **"Eye hath not seen, nor ear heard, nor entered into the heart of man the things that the Lord has prepared for them that love Him."** I Cor. 2:9

I must say again that in my wildest imagination, after reading passages in the Word, and hearing sermons and songs about Heaven all my life, I could never have grasped the concept of the beauty and peace that exists there. My finite mind could never have conceived the reality of golden streets and shiny pearly gates! To be in the presence of Jesus was indescribable. I must repeat it was awe-inspiring! He stood before me glowing with majesty and I felt a sense of power unknown in the natural world we are born into. There isn't any place on earth where one could travel and see what I was seeing at that moment.

Jesus is the focal point, the centerpiece of all activity. I fell at His feet to worship Him. He lifted my face toward Him and in the most gentle, yet authoritative voice I've ever heard said, "*Daughter, enter into the joy of your everlasting inheritance.*"

DON'T CRY

Don't cry for me or weep and carry on

for I am in a better land
where you, too, soon shall come.

Do not mourn. Let rejoicing be, for now I'm free!
Free from life's struggle for health and for gain,
perfect in Jesus whose name I proclaim!

Heaven's beauty overwhelms me
so vast and so grand.
Oh, how God loves us to include us in His plan.

Angelic host a choir compose
and loud hosannas ring,
giving honor to our Lord: He is the King of Kings!

Don't cry for me or weep and carry on
for I am in a better land
where you, too, soon shall come!

THE PROMISE OF IMMORTALITY

(Excerpts from I Corinthians 15)

"So also is the resurrection of the dead. It is sown in corruption; it is raised in incorruption; it is sown in dishonor; it is raised in glory; it is sown in weakness; it is raised in power;

"It is sown a natural body; it is raised a spiritual body. There is a natural body and there is a spiritual body. And as we have borne the image of the earthly, we shall also bear the image of the heavenly. Now this I say, brethren, that flesh and blood cannot inherit the kingdom of God; neither doth corruption inherit incorruption.

"Behold, I show you a mystery; we shall not all sleep, but we shall be changed in a moment, in the twinkling of an eye, at the last trump: for the trumpet will sound and the dead shall be raised incorruptible, and we shall be changed.

"For this corruptible must put on incorruption and this mortal must put on immortality. So when this corruptible shall have put on incorruption, and this mortal shall have put on immortality, then shall be brought to pass the saying that is written, 'Death is swallowed up in victory.'

"Oh death, where is thy sting? O grave, where is thy victory? The sting of death is sin and the sting of sin is the law. But thanks be to God, who gives us the victory through our Lord Jesus Christ."

PART TWO

We All Need a Savior

This section is primarily for readers who have never made a decision to receive Jesus Christ as their Savior and they would like to do so now. It's not at all complicated. We become children of God through faith in Him.

BACKGROUND

In the beginning of time God created the heavens and the earth, everything was perfect. There was no sin. God created man and woman and placed them in the beautiful Garden of Eden. The garden was lush with vines and bushes as well as fruit-bearing trees. God and man walked and talked together in the Garden every day.

God told Adam and Eve they could eat of all the trees in the beautiful garden except one. They were not to eat of the Tree of Knowledge of Good and Evil. They must have discussed this between them. One day the sly serpent tempted Eve to eat of the forbidden fruit. "You shall not die," he said. "Take a bite and see if you die. Surely God didn't really mean you would die if you eat of the forbidden fruit." The serpent made it sound so good and the fruit on the tree was most tempting.

Finally, Eve couldn't resist. She plucked fruit from the tree and took a bite. She had never tasted such wonderful flavor. It was sweet and juicy, absolutely wonderful! She offered a bite to Adam. He saw the look of contentment on Eve's face and couldn't resist her offer of the forbidden fruit. This was the first act of disobedience to God.

As a result of their sin, God put them, the first man and woman, out of the garden. The sin of disobedience had separated them from walking and talking directly to God. Though they did not fall down and die a physical death, they experienced separation from God, their creator. This was spiritual death.
Genesis 2:16,17

Many years later the Messiah was born in Bethlehem as was prophesied in the Old Testament. Isaiah 9:6 reads:
".....a child will be born to us, a Son will be given to us. And the government will rest on His shoulders; and His name shall be called Wonderful Counselor, Mighty God, Eternal Father, Prince of Peace."

The promised Savior came to earth in humble surroundings of a lowly manger. He matured and became a miracle worker and healer as He walked the shores of Galilee. (Read the account of His birth in Luke.)

Jesus spoke with authority in the temple. Throngs of people flocked to His side. Religious leaders accused Him of blasphemy because He declared Himself to be the Son of God. The chief priests feared Jesus would take their following away They did not have power to heal the afflicted and feed thousands on a hillside with only a few fish and a little bread as they had seen Him do. They plotted to kill Jesus. Satan entered into one of the disciples who delivered Jesus to his accusers as He prayed in Gethsemane.

A crown of thorns was pressed angrily upon His head and blood ran down His face. He was spit upon and ridiculed. The angry, jealous mob removed his robe and severely beat him on the back. They nailed his hands and feet to a rugged, wooden cross and thrust a spear into His side. The Son of God hung between heaven and earth, the ultimate sacrifice for your sins and mine.

Jesus had told His disciples He would rise from the grave on the third day. His body was placed into a tomb and sealed securely by centurions. Guards were placed to make certain nobody would come in the dead of night and steal Jesus' body away. Amazingly, those in power thought they could entomb Jesus and make the grave secure by placing a two-ton rock over the entrance.

On the third day, as Jesus had promised, **He arose from the grave** in the most unusual of circumstances. There was a great earthquake. The astonished guards trembled at the event. The sealed tomb was opened! The rock at the entrance of the tomb was rolled away. The tomb was empty; Jesus was not there. He was triumphant over death. The guards proclaimed, "Truly this was the Son of God!"

Later Jesus revealed Himself to His disciples who saw the nail prints in His hands, witness that He truly was the risen Savior. DO YOU KNOW OF AN EVENT SUCH AS THIS WHEN ONE WHO WAS PROCLAIMED DEAD AND BURIED CAME BACK TO LIFE? NO YOU DON'T.

THERE HAS NEVER BEEN ANOTHER HISTORICAL EVENT WHEN ANYONE WAS BURIED IN A TOMB AND STEPPED FORTH IN RESURRECTION POWER, LEAVING GRAVE CLOTHES FOLDED NEATLY INSIDE. Because Jesus rose from the dead, all who believe in Him have hope of eternal life when they repent of their sins and receive Him as Savior. The Bible teaches us, "To be absent from the body is to be present with the Lord."

When our earthly shell expires, our souls are transported into God's presence. What a glorious time that will be for Christians! We will never suffer pain, loss or failure again. Oh how God loves us to give His only begotten Son as the supreme sacrifice for the sins of man.

It is a privilege to serve Him. How can anyone resist the love of God who has made a way for us to escape damnation and inherit eternal life?

BASIC SALVATION SCRIPTURES:
"For all have sinned and come short the glory of God." Romans 3:23

"For the wages of sin is death, but the gift of God is eternal life through Jesus Christ our Lord."
Romans 6:23

"For this purpose the Son of God was manifest that He might destroy the works of the devil." I John 3:8

"For God so loved the world that He gave His only begotten son that whosoever believeth in Him should not perish, but have eternal life." John 3:16

"If we confess our sins, He is faithful and just to forgive our sins and cleanse us from all unrighteousness." I John 1:9

HOW DO I BECOME A CHRISTIAN?

Becoming a Christian is not at all complicated. The first step in becoming a Christian is to recognize you are a sinner. Confess your sins directly to God, through prayer. Ask Him to forgive your sins and He will make you clean. You may pray a simple prayer, such as, "Jesus I am a sinner who needs your forgiveness. I know you died on the cross for me, taking the penalty for my sin. I now receive you as my Savior and I will live for you all the days of my life. Thank you for the hope I have of eternal life through your shed blood on the cross."

WHAT DO I DO NOW?

A Christian is a *follower of Jesus Christ.* As a follower of Christ you will want to know who Christ is and what He has taught us to do. How do we learn more about

Jesus Christ? By reading the Word of God commonly referred to as The Holy Bible. If you don't have a Bible in your home, they are readily available in local bookstores or thrift stores. When you find a church to attend, ask the pastor for a Bible. He'll be thrilled to provide one for you.

Some of you may be too ill to hold a Bible for reading. If you have that difficulty, there are Bible CD's or DVD's readily available. Possibly an acquaintance has the Bible on DVD and would allow you to borrow it. Don't be too timid to ask. Further, you can always ask someone to read the Bible to you.

FELLOWSHIP

One cannot emphasize enough the value of Christian fellowship. You'll find fellowship in a local church. This is where godly pastors deliver the Word of God with dynamic authority. Fellowship with other believers is an essential part of Christian growth. Look for an evangelical church where Jesus is acknowledged as the Son of God, the Savior. Become acquainted with the pastor; let him know of your terminal illness so he may pray for you.

Pastors are God's gracious gift to the church to teach, encourage and guide believers. They want to be a blessing and source of inspiration – this is their calling. Don't hesitate to counsel with the man of God.

174

As a new believer in Jesus Christ the road of life isn't going to immediately be smooth sailing. There will be trials along the way. Indeed, you will have struggles, but these are the things that make us grow and mature in the Lord. Trials of life cannot smother the new joy you have found in serving the Lord.

Remember, too, you are afflicted with a serious disease from which you may not be a survivor, so you want to learn how to pray (speaking directly with God). You also want to know who Jesus is. If you are able, read the four gospels of Matthew, Mark, Luke and John. Here you will see Jesus in action when he walked the shores of Galilee.

The New Testament has much to say about living a life in Christ Jesus. Take time each day to pray. If you need deliverance from sinful habits such as cursing, lust, pornography, drugs, sexual sins, etc., He will give you strength to overcome the temptation to sin. Sinful habits may also delay healing for your body; a change in life style may be what you need.

You'll soon discover the Lord is always near to hear your prayer and give you guidance. He speaks to us through His Word and also through our thoughts or by strong impressions.

"He who overcomes shall inherit all things, and I will be His God and he shall be My son. But the coward-

ly, unbelieving, murderers, sexually immoral, sorcerers, idolaters, and all liars shall have their part in the lake which burns with fire and brimstone......"
Rev. 21:7,8

"My little children, these things write I unto you that you sin not. And if any man sins we have an advocate with the Father, Jesus Christ......" I John 2:1

An advocate is someone who goes before the Judge to intercede on another's behalf. Isn't it wonderful to know that Jesus is your advocate, interceding on your behalf before Father God? Oh, how He loves you! When you sin you need to (1) recognize it; (2) ask the Lord for forgiveness and (3) make an effort not to repeat the sin again. God bless you as you begin your new life in Jesus Christ.

If the Lord should choose to call you home you will be sheltered in the arms of God. You will spend eternity in Heaven where there is no sin, no sadness, only pure exhilaration to be in the presence of Almighty God. YOU NOW ENJOY EVERLASTING LIFE!

When you step from Earth to Glory, you will surely say, *"It has been worth it all."*

**What a blessed day
that will be for all of us
when we see Jesus!**

Declaration of Faith

I hereby testify that after careful consideration of scripture and by the prompting of the Holy Spirit I now receive Jesus Christ as my Savior.

Having repented of my sins, I shall endeavor to walk worthy of the calling of God.

_____

Name

_____

Date

You are hereby welcomed into the fellowship of born again Christians worldwide.

www.ingramcontent.com/pod-product-compliance
Lightning Source LLC
Chambersburg PA
CBHW062204280526

45788CB00001B/438